A Colour Handbook

Gastroenterology
Second edition

Ralph Boulton
PhD, FRCP

Consultant Gastroenterologist, Department of Gastroenterology
University Hospital Birmingham NHS Foundation Trust, Birmingham, UK

Claire Cousins
FRCP, FRCR

Consultant Radiologist, Department of Radiology, Addenbrooke's Hospital
Cambridge University Hospitals NHS Foundation Trust, Cambridge, UK

Sanjeev Gupta
MBBS, MD, FRCP

Professor of Medicine and Pathology, Eleazar and Feige Reicher Chair in Translational Medicine,
Divisions of Hepatology and Gastroenterology and Nutrition, Albert Einstein College of Medicine,
Bronx NY, USA

Humphrey Hodgson
F Med Sci, FRCP

Sheila Sherlock Chair of Medicine, Director, Centre for Hepatology Royal Free/Hampstead
University College School of Medicine, London, UK

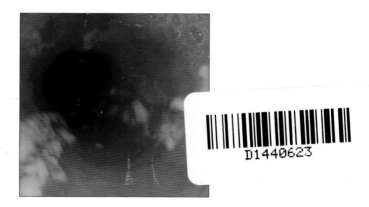

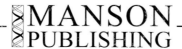

MANSON
PUBLISHING

For full details of all Manson Publishing titles please write to:
Manson Publishing Ltd, 73 Corringham Road, London NW11 7DL, UK.
Tel: +44(0)20 8905 5150
Fax: +44(0)20 8201 9233
Website: www.mansonpublishing.com

Commissioning editor: Jill Northcott
Project manager: Julie Bennett
Copy editor: Janet E. Tosh
Proof reader: Carrie Walker
Layout: DiacriTech, India
Colour reproduction: Tenon & Polert Colour Scanning Ltd, Hong Kong
Printed by: Finidr, s.r.o., Cesky Tesin, Czech Republic

CONTENTS

PREFACE

The speciality of gastroenterology continues to evolve. New imaging technology, refinements in endoscopy, development of new therapy, and the onward creep of scientific knowledge all contribute to this. To continue dealing with the range of diseases encompassed by gastroenterology, practising clinicians must assimilate these changes into their day-to-day work. Nevertheless, gastroenterology remains a very attractive and practical speciality. The aim of this book is to convey the continued excitement of practising this area of medicine.

This second edition is still aimed at trainees. In an era when junior doctors need to make career choices at an early stage of postgraduate training, the book aims to serve as a solid introduction to the field of gastroenterology.

The second edition retains the familiar format of a concise overview of the major pathologies, each linked with key images. In the age of the internet, with such ready access to information, this organization of the material should continue to assist in the learning of gastroenterology, and to help in the evaluation of information from these other sources.

Ralph Boulton

ACKNOWLEDGEMENTS

We are grateful to a number of our colleagues for providing illustrative material, either with material from their own collection, or because their expertise allowed the procedures to be performed in the first instance. These include Dr James Jackson, Professor John Calam, Dr Julian Walters, Dr Simon Taylor-Robinson, Mr John Spencer, Mr Witold Kmiot, Dr AJW Hilson, Dr Shirley Hodgson, Mr Mohammed Aslam, Dr Simon Olliff, Dr N de Souza, Professor Michael Peters, Dr Brin Mahon, Ms Joanne Hayes, Dr Peter Guest, Dr Iqbal Khan, Dr Philipe Taniere, Dr Ian McCafferty, Dr Mark Narain, Mr Simon Radley, Dr John Lee, Dr Jeff Butterworth, Dr Martin Toy, Dr Kam Mangat, Dr Shri Pathmakanthan, Dr Douglas Thorburn, Dr Kate Kane, Mr Darius Mirza, Dr Andrew Robinson, Professor Dion Morton, Dr Andrew Latchford, Dr Rupert Ransford, and Dr Peter Riley.

We would also like to thank Dr Roy Cockel, University Hospital Birmingham NHS Foundation Trust, for allowing us to publish some of his endoscopic images.

Finally, we acknowledge Cambridge Life Sciences Ltd (Endosc–HP urease test), Given Imaging Ltd (wireless capsule endoscopy system), Synectics Medical Ltd and University Hospital Birmingham library.

CONTRIBUTORS

Ralph Boulton PhD FRCP
Consultant Gastroenterologist
Department of Gastroenterology
University Hospital Birmingham NHS
    Foundation Trust
Birmingham B29 6JD

Humphrey Hodgson F Med Sci FRCP
Sheila Sherlock Chair of Medicine
Director, Centre for Hepatology Royal
    Free/Hampstead
University College School of Medicine
Rowland Hill Street
London NW3 2PF

Claire Cousins FRCP, FRCR
Consultant Radiologist
Department of Radiology Box 218
Addenbrooke's Hospital
Cambridge University Hospitals NHS
    Foundation Trust
Hills Road
Cambridge CB2 0QQ

Sanjeev Gupta, MBBS, MD, FRCP
Professor of Medicine and Pathology
Eleazar and Feige Reicher Chair in
    Translational Medicine
Divisions of Hepatology and Gastroenterology
    and Nutrition
Albert Einstein College of Medicine
Ullmann Building, Room 625
1300 Morris Park Avenue
Bronx NY 10461, USA

ABBREVIATIONS

AIDS	acquired immunodeficiency syndrome
ALT	alanine aminotransferase
ANCA	antineutrophil cytoplasmic antibody
APACHE	Acute Physiology and Chronic Health Evaluation
APC	adenomatous polyposis coli
APUD	amine precursor uptake and decarboxylation
5-ASA	5-amino-salicylic acid
AST	aspartate aminotransferase
CEA	carcinoembryonic antigen
CF	cystic fibrosis
CFTR	cystic fibrosis transmembrane conductance regulator
CHRPE	congenital hypertrophy of the retinal pigment epithelium
CMV	cytomegalovirus
CNS	central nervous system
CRP	C-reactive protein
CT	computed tomography
DALM	dysplasia-associated lesion or mass
DCC	deleted in colon carcinoma
DEXA	dual energy X-ray absorptiometry
EATL	enteropathy associated T-cell lymphoma
EBV	Epstein–Barr virus
EGFR	epidermal growth factor receptor
ELISA	enzyme-linked immunosorbent assay
ERC	endoscopic retrograde cholangiography
ERCP	endoscopic retrograde cholangiopancreatography
ESR	erythrocyte sedimentation rate
EUS	endoscopic ultrasound
FAP	familial adenomatous polyposis
GGT	gamma-glutamyltransferase
GISTs	gastrointestinal stromal tumours
GORD	gastro-oesophageal reflux disease
GRF	growth hormone-releasing factor
HHT	hereditary haemorrhagic telangiectasia
5-HIAA	5-hydroxy-indole acetic acid
HIDA	(2, 6-diethylacetanilide)-iminodiacetic acid
HIV	human immunodeficiency virus
HLA	human leukocyte antigen
HNPCC	hereditary nonpolyposis colorectal cancer
HPV	human papilloma virus
HSV	herpes simplex virus
ITU	intensive therapy unit
IV	intravenous
LDH	lactate dehydrogenase
LEDs	light-emitting diodes
LOS	lower oesophageal sphincter
MALTomas	mucosa-associated lymphoid tissue lymphomas
MCV	mean corpuscular volume
MEN	multiple endocrine neoplasia
6-MP	6-mercaptopurine
MR	magnetic resonance
MRC	magnetic resonance cholangiography
MRCP	magnetic resonance cholangiopancreatography
MRI	magnetic resonance imaging
NSAIDs	nonsteroidal anti-inflammatory drugs
PABA	para-aminobenzoic acid
PAS	periodic acid–Schiff
PCR	polymerase chain reaction
PET	positron-emission tomography
PLE	protein-losing enteropathy
PP	pancreatic polypeptide
PSC	primary sclerosing cholangitits
PTC	percutaneous transhepatic cholangiography
SBDS	Shwachman–Bodian–Diamond syndrome
SGS	short gut syndrome
SSRI	selective serotonin reuptake inhibitor
STK	serine threonine kinase
TIPSS	transjugular intrahepatic portosystemic shunt
tTG	tissue transglutaminase
VEGF	vascular endothelial growth factor
VIP	vasoactive intestinal peptide
WBC	white blood cell count

CHAPTER 1

Gastroenterological problems

Elicit an accurate history

Examine the patient

Gastroenterological disease can cause systemic symptoms

Systemic disease can cause gastroenterological symptoms

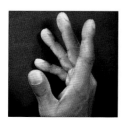 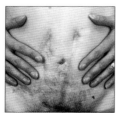 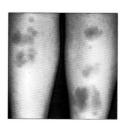 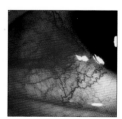

Introduction

Gastroenterological problems encompass the entire range of pathology, including neoplasm, infection, inflammation, immunological disorders, biochemical, metabolic and congenital conditions, and disorders of unknown cause. In addition, approximately one-third of the gastrointestinal symptoms of outpatients have no identifiable structural, infective, or biochemical disorder present – they appear as 'functional disorders'. Within such disorders, psychological or social factors may be primarily responsible. Identification and correct management depends on accurate history taking, clinical examination, and specialist investigations.

Approach to the patient

Some cardinal symptoms focus attention on one particular organ, and dictate the most effective and economical investigational path. Be aware that some disease processes outside the abdomen may present with abdominal symptoms, and consider the patient as a whole.

Major presenting complaints

DIFFICULTY IN SWALLOWING (DYSPHAGIA)

Difficulty in transferring food from the mouth to the stomach is termed dysphagia. This is an important symptom and it is useful to distinguish between the two phases of the normal swallow. The initial oropharyngeal phase, during which a food bolus is moved from the mouth to the oesophagus, is under voluntary control. This is followed by the oesophageal phase, which is involuntary.

Difficulty in starting the swallow – oropharyngeal dysphagia

This relates to neurological or muscular diseases (bulbar, pseudobulbar palsy, motor neurone disease, myasthenia gravis). It is often associated with drooling due to difficulty in swallowing saliva, or aspiration of saliva and aspiration pneumonia. There may be associated problems with voice production.

Food sticking after swallowing has started – oesophageal dysphagia

This suggests the presence of a structural lesion in the oesophagus. Some patients can actually localize the level of food sticking, while others cannot.

The nature of food that elicits symptoms should be clarified. Dysphagia initially for liquids is more likely to reflect problems in muscular or neural control of swallowing. Dysphagia initially for solids is likely to reflect a structural lesion in the oesophagus. Progressive dysphagia, first for solids, then for sloppy food and liquids, is a sinister sign that is strongly suggestive of cancer of the oesophagus, although this can occur with peptic strictures from recurrent oesophagitis.

Nonprogressive dysphagia may suggest a benign structural lesion (e.g. mucosal web in upper oesophagus, benign 'ring' in lower oesophagus). Intermittent food sticking, affecting both solids and liquids, suggests disordered motility (achalasia, oesophageal spasm).

With any oesophageal obstruction, regurgitation of food and liquid into the mouth may occur. The fluid is bland and not bitter, as it does not contain gastric acid. Nocturnal regurgitation may be associated with choking, aspiration, pneumonia, or asthma.

Lump in throat (globus hystericus or globus sensation)

During stress, highly anxious individuals may complain of a sensation of a lump in the throat without having eaten or drunk, often with temporary inability to swallow. This is a temporary functional disorder associated with anxiety. It is more common in women and, although investigations are frequently normal, it is sometimes associated with other oesophageal conditions (reflux disease and motility disorders). Gastropharyngeal reflux accounts for the symptoms in some.

LOSS OF APPETITE

This is highly nonspecific, but may be functional if associated with anxiety or depression. When associated with weight loss, it suggests significant organic disease. A maintained appetite is a reassuring sign that serious disease is less likely to be found. Early satiety (initial hunger but a rapid feeling of fullness after commencing eating) may reflect a poorly distensible stomach or a motility disorder.

NAUSEA AND VOMITING

These are nonspecific symptoms. In young men, morning nausea and retching without vomiting strongly suggests alcoholism. In young women, morning nausea suggests pregnancy. Nausea occurs with many abdominal pains, particularly those reflecting spasm of smooth muscle. Examples include an obstructed biliary tract, or spasm of the colon in functional bowel disease. Vomiting is a more significant disturbance involving reverse peristalsis and expulsion of gastric contents. It is rare as a purely functional disorder, although in a few patients 'hysterical vomiting' is the final diagnosis, generally reflecting severe family stress. More often, vomiting reflects organic disease affecting the stomach, duodenum, or small intestine.

Short-lived vomiting with fever and diarrhoea suggests food poisoning (bacteria, bacterial toxins, viral gastroenteritis).

Prolonged vomiting over more than a few days needs further investigation. In the absence of pain, persistent vomiting suggests obstruction of the outflow tract of the stomach, as seen with antral carcinoma or narrowing of the pylorus due to long-standing duodenal ulceration.

The nature of vomitus may be significant. Vomiting food ingested many hours previously suggests obstruction of the gastric outlet, as the stomach normally empties within 4–6 hr of eating. Vomiting of blood is discussed below.

Vomiting must be distinguished from regurgitation (food returning to mouth from gullet without reverse peristalsis), and from waterbrash (the mouth filled with salty water due to excess saliva, sometimes a symptom of peptic ulceration).

Both vomiting and nausea can reflect events elsewhere in the body (e.g. raised intracranial pressure, severe metabolic complications such as renal failure, side effects of drugs). Prolonged vomiting can induce metabolic changes, for example hypokalaemic alkalosis and secondary potassium loss from the kidneys.

PAIN

This is the most common reason for referral to gastroenterologists. Classic symptom complexes are sometimes recognizable, but some pains are poorly characterized and localized. The site and radiation of pain should be defined, and its duration (minutes or hours) noted. Pain character should also be noted – is the pain sharp, dull, or intermittent? Periodicity details should be noted – whether pain occurs all day, occasionally but every day, or every day for some weeks and then not at all for some months, is important diagnostically. Timing and relationship of pain to eating, defaecation, and sleep should be noted. Relieving factors should be elucidated, and associated symptoms elicited (e.g. vomiting, nausea, weight loss). Major patterns of pain are described below.

Heartburn (pyrosis)

This is best reserved to describe sensations that occur when gastric acid refluxes into the oesophagus, but patients use the term in different contexts. There is a raw burning sensation, retrosternally, lasting for some minutes, which may start in the epigastrium and travel back to the throat. Heartburn is precipitated by large meals, alcohol, stooping, or lying flat in bed. It is rapidly relieved by drinking milk/alkali. Persistent severe heartburn suggests the presence of oesophagitis (inflammation in the oesophagus) and repeated reflux. When severe, dysphagia may result. The condition may eventually be complicated by stricture. Reflux is often, but not invariably, associated with hiatus hernia.

Dyspepsia

Epigastric pain altered by food intake is the classical symptom of peptic ulceration. Symptoms of duodenal and gastric ulceration, duodenitis, and gastritis all overlap and are not distinguishable without investigation. Often, epigastric discomfort related to food is associated with negative findings on further examination, particularly in anxious patients. The classical duodenal ulcer history is epigastric pain, which is relieved by food and brought on by hunger; the pain is epigastric or radiating through to the back. Antacids relieve symptoms usually within minutes. The pain often wakes the patient in the early hours. Symptoms may come in bouts (daily for several weeks and then remitting for months or years). Associated nausea and vomiting may be prominent with gastric ulcers or prepyloric ulcers.

Gallbladder and biliary pain

Pain from the biliary tract reflects either spasm of smooth muscle or acute inflammation. Spasm is due to obstruction of the common bile duct or the neck of the gallbladder, usually by a gallstone. The full-blown syndrome of biliary colic is unmistakable – severe right upper quadrant pain, radiating laterally to the back, in waves superimposed on a severe discomfort. This lasts for several hours, generally with nausea and vomiting. Patients classically roam around to find a comfortable position. An inflamed gallbladder (cholecystitis) gives similar sited pain, though it is more likely to radiate to the shoulder. Minor discomfort is attributed to postprandial contraction of the gallbladder (right upper quadrant discomfort, excessive belching, nausea) but these are often nonspecific.

Pancreatic pain

Chronic inflammation gives severe pain in the back just below the shoulder blades, brought about by eating or alcohol, and mildly relieved by leaning forward. This history is also compatible with duodenal ulceration. Much pancreatic pain is ill-defined – dyspepsia affecting the epigastrium, or right or left side of the abdomen, and with an indefinite relationship to food. Pancreatic cancer may be painless, but extension retroperitoneally initiates unremitting central back pain.

Intestinal pain

Normal peristalsis is painless. Short-lived, acute painful peristalsis – intestinal colic – is readily recognized, usually due to acute gastroenteritis. Repeated or persistent painful peristalsis generally indicates intestinal narrowing or obstruction, most commonly due to adhesions and previous surgery or tumours. There is intermittent sharp exacerbation of pain, doubling up the patient when pain is severe. The full-blown picture of complete obstruction is a constellation of crampy pains, distension, borborygmi (audible, high-pitched bowel sounds), nausea, and eventually failure to pass bowel motions or flatus.

Small-intestinal colic is poorly localized but predominantly central and above the umbilicus. Colonic colic is characteristically low in the abdomen, below the umbilicus, and is relieved by defaecation. Intestinal inflammation can be painful. Transmural inflammation with secondary inflammation of parietal peritoneum, e.g. appendicitis, gives well-localized pain over the inflamed organ, but is worse on movement or prodding.

Severe acute abdominal pain

A number of rare causes should be considered in addition to classical surgical emergencies of obstruction or perforation. Consider coronary artery insufficiency (angina or myocardial infarction can be epigastric). Aortic disease – dissection, aneurysm, or dilatation – may give epigastric pain. Intestinal ischaemia can cause recurrent noncolicky pain induced by eating, with characteristic weight loss as food is avoided due to fear of pain. Metabolic disorders (acute intermittent porphyria) comprise a rare but important cause.

BLEEDING

Gut bleeding varies from acute and life-threatening, to chronic and trivial. Most bleeding comes from the upper gastrointestinal tract, presenting either with haematemesis and melaena, or just melaena. The source is variable, from oesophagus to upper jejunum. Lower gastrointestinal haemorrhage is less common as an emergency, and varies from trivial haemorrhoids (bright red bleeding on toilet paper after defaecation) to more severe causes – cancer, polyps, diverticular disease and vascular malformation, or inflammatory colitis in association with diarrhoea. Bleeding from the distal colon is normally fairly bright red, but from the caecum is plum-coloured or darker. Low-grade chronic blood loss may be invisible (occult) and present with anaemia.

ABNORMAL BOWEL HABIT

Normal bowel habit varies between people, from two or three loose stools daily to hard motions every second or third day. Changes in pre-existing pattern are more significant than long-standing deviation from what the patient or doctor considers 'normal'.

Constipation

This is described as infrequent passage of stools, which become dehydrated and hard from a long stay in the colon (see Chapter 10). Trivial causes include immobility, diminished food intake, and medication with constipating agents, e.g. codeine. Constipation requires further investigation when recent in origin or associated with colicky pain.

Diarrhoea

This requires careful definition. Diarrhoea may describe states from moderate to frequent passage of formed stools, to massive volumes of liquid stool. Many patients with a 'diarrhoeal' form of irritable bowel have two to three loose motions in the morning, usually after food, but the total mass of stool is normal. Diarrhoea waking a patient at night is generally significant. Passage of blood and mucus is obviously significant, but passage of mucus alone does not indicate pathology. Clinical indications of steatorrhoea (pale, floating, foul-smelling) (1) are unreliable indicators of excess fat (malabsorption). Observation of rainbow colours on the surface of the stool or lavatory pan water implies severe steatorrhoea – such as seen in pancreatic insufficiency or extensive resection of the small gut. Inflammatory colitis, or ischaemic change in the colon, is often associated with crampy abdominal colic, but disease of the small intestine can also cause colonic colic as excess fluid enters the colon. Under normal circumstances, less than 1.25 l of intestinal fluid leaves the ileum to enter the colon, which then reduces the volume to less than 300 ml. Liquid stool volumes of more than 1.5 l a day, therefore, strongly suggest disease of the small gut.

RECTAL SYMPTOMS

Symptoms from the rectum include:
- Tenesmus: this refers to a feeling of rectal fullness and a sensation that the bowel needs evacuation (even if a bowel motion has recently been passed). It reflects the presence of rectal inflammation.
- Constant anal pain (suggesting the presence of an abscess or thrombosed haemorrhoid).
- A tearing pain on defaecation (suggesting an anal fissure).
- Proctalgia fugax: an intense intermittent anal pain attributed to spasm.
- Pruritus ani: anal itch, which occurs idiopathically or in the presence of pinworm infection.

WEIGHT LOSS

In combination with other gastrointestinal symptoms, this is a major symptom. Systemic conditions (thyrotoxicosis, tuberculosis, diabetes, cancer, and anxiety) should also be considered.

OTHER GASTROINTESTINAL SYMPTOMS

Other less well-defined complaints should be considered. Abdominal distension, particularly after meals, is one classical manifestation of functional bowel disease, probably reflecting delayed emptying of small-intestinal contents into the caecum. Other symptoms include alternation between constipation and diarrhoea, colicky colonic pain, and intermittent discomfort in the right upper quadrant, left upper quadrant, or left lower quadrant of the abdomen. Long-standing symptoms in the presence of otherwise good health, dating back many years, or persistent abnormality of bowel habit following an acute attack of gastroenteritis, are suggestive clinical features for diagnosis of irritable bowel syndrome.

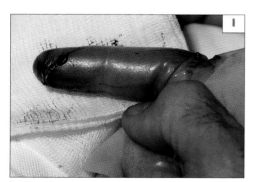

1 'Silver stool' – the pale steatorrhoeic stool, together with the presence of altered blood, in a patient with a combination of obstructive jaundice and bleeding into the gut.

Functional gastrointestinal syndromes

Many patients present with symptoms that seem to arise from the gastrointestinal tract, but for which no specific structural explanation is apparent. These are termed functional gastrointestinal syndromes. They are common in the general population and account for a large proportion of new referrals to gastrointestinal outpatient clinics. Typically, there are other symptoms in other systems, for example gynaecological symptoms or fibromyalgia. As a group, patients score highly in indices of depression and anxiety, although individual patients do not usually meet the criteria for formal psychiatric diagnosis.

IRRITABLE BOWEL SYNDROME
Definition
Irritable bowel syndrome is characterized by chronic abdominal pain, associated with an altered bowel habit in the absence of an organic cause.

Epidemiology
There is a common constellation of symptoms, reported by around 20% of the general population in surveys. However, most sufferers do not seek medical attention. The disease is mostly diagnosed in young adults, and more frequently in women (female:male 2:1). Familial clustering has been noted in some studies, either representing heritable pathophysiological changes or an environmental contributor.

Aetiology
The aetiology of irritable bowel syndrome is not known. There are a number of theories, including changes in visceral pain perception, alteration of motility, and bacterial overgrowth. Frequently, patients give a history of an antecedent infective gastroenteritis. Psychological dysfunction (typically anxiety, depression, and somatization) is over-represented in patients referred to tertiary care centres, but is insufficient to meet criteria for formal psychiatric diagnosis.

Clinical features
The features of irritable bowel syndrome are variable and frequently fluctuate. There may be a history of diarrhoea or constipation, or alternation between these patterns. Abdominal pain tends to accompany the changes in bowel habit. Features such as rectal bleeding, nocturnal symptoms, or systemic symptoms such as weight loss should lead to a consideration of other diagnoses.

Management
A proactive approach to making the diagnosis with the minimum of investigation is better than making irritable bowel syndrome a diagnosis of exclusion. Careful and reassuring explanations of the benign nature of the condition are frequently helpful.

Drug therapy
This is led by the dominant symptoms. Diarrhoea is treated with antidiarrhoeal drugs such as loperamide. Antispasmodic drugs are frequently prescribed, although there is little evidence of efficacy. Low-dose tricyclic antidepressants are used particularly for abdominal pain, and seem to have an action independent of anxiety or depression. Global symptom improvement has been reported with selective serotonin reuptake inhibitors (SSRIs).

Physical examination of the gastroenterology patient

The historical features outlined above will have suggested a short differential diagnosis. In many patients with gastrointestinal disease, no abnormal physical findings will be demonstrable. Nonetheless, a physical examination, which should not be confined to the abdomen, should be made. Aspects of the general physical examination that may provide useful clues to gastroenterological and hepatic conditions are given in *Table 1* (**2–8**, overleaf).

LIVER

An enlarged, tender liver may be inflamed, congested, or the site of an abscess or tumour. The patency of the hepatic venous drainage can be checked by showing elevation of the jugular venous pressure on pressing over the liver. Although a crude physical sign, there is a good correlation between the finding of a fibrous, hard liver and cirrhosis. Rapid changes in liver size may indicate mobilization of fat, and in alcoholic patients the liver may diminish in size rapidly on abstention from alcohol. A hepatic bruit may be heard in alcoholic hepatitis or in patients with tumours.

Table 1 General physical signs of gastrointestinal disease

Hands

Liver palms	Acute or chronic liver disease
Clubbing (**2, 3**)	Cirrhosis, Crohn's disease
Leukonychia (white nails)	Liver disease, protein-losing enteropathy
Dupuytren's contracture	Alcoholism

Skin

Spider naevi	Cirrhosis or hepatitis
White spots	Chronic liver disease (**4**)
Pigmentation (**4**)	Haemochromatosis, internal malignancy, malabsorption
Blisters, depigmentation	Porphryia cutanea tarda
Erythema nodosum (**5**)	Inflammatory bowel disease

Eyes

Coloration	Jaundice (**6**)
Episcleritis (**7**)/iritis	Inflammatory bowel disease (**3**)
Retinal appearances	Pseudoxanthoma elasticum
Venous pressure	Hepatic pain in congestive cardiac failure
	Cardiological causes of ascites or protein-losing enteropathy
Lymphadenopathy	Carcinoma of the stomach and other malignancies
Cyanosis	Severe liver disease
Anaemia	Acute and chronic gastrointestinal blood loss
Cardiac disease and peripheral pulses	Intestinal angina, ischaemic gut disease, mesenteric emboli
Gynaecomastia	Chronic liver disease
Peripheral neuropathy	Alcoholism, amyloidosis, porphyria, vitamin B_{12} deficiency due to malabsorption
Encephalopathy	Liver disease
Erythema *ab igne* (**8**)	Chronic pain
(mottled pigmentation of the skin due to application of external heat)	

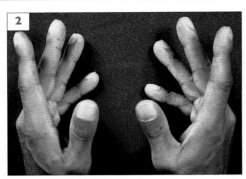

2 Clubbing of the fingers.

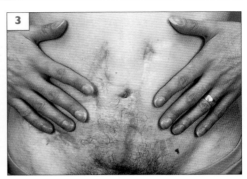

3 Clubbing and multiple scars point to chronic inflammatory bowel disease.

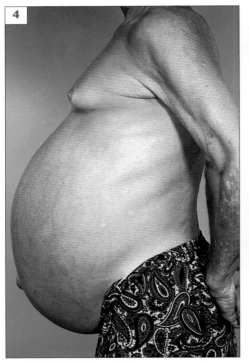

4 Gynaecomastia, ascites, and pigmentation all point to chronic liver disease in this patient.

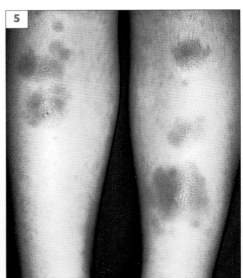

5 Erythema nodosum, seen in Crohn's disease or ulcerative colitis.

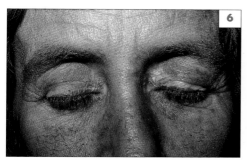

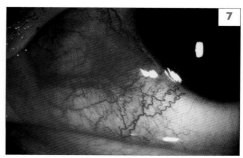

6 Jaundice; xanthelasma around the eyes in chronic cholestatic jaundice (primary biliary cirrhosis).

7 Episcleritis, another association of active inflammatory bowel disease.

8 Erythema *ab igne*, due to applied heat in an attempt to relieve chronic pain in a patient with a narrow terminal ileum causing recurrent abdominal pain.

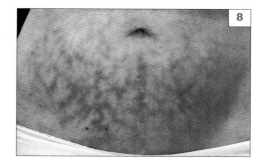

SPLEEN

Palpating the spleen can be difficult. Rotating the patient on to the right side, a helping examiner's hand on the left flank, and deep inspiration may all make the examination easier.

ASCITES

While gross ascites is easy to detect (**4, 333**), one may be misled into diagnosing ascites in gross obesity, as fat is liquid at body temperature. Minor degrees of ascites can be difficult to detect clinically, but ultrasound examination will settle any doubt.

ABDOMINAL BRUITS

Bruits in the epigastrium are not necessarily pathological, as the superior mesenteric artery may often be stretched over the pancreas. Nonetheless, they should lead to consideration of a diagnosis of intestinal ischaemia or a pancreatic tumour.

HERNIAL ORIFICES, SCARS

Hernial orifices and scars are relevant in the context of colicky abdominal pain, as they may indicate obstruction in the hernial sac or the presence of adhesions.

Mouth and pharynx

Examining the mouth may show signs suggestive of gastrointestinal disease

The appearances of the tongue can reflect vitamin deficiencies

Mouth ulcers may reflect coeliac disease or Crohn's disease

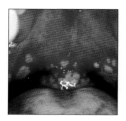
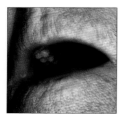
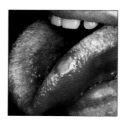
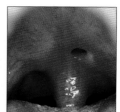

Oral problems

The mouth is the most easily examined part of the gastrointestinal tract. Important clues to systemic illness, and to disease elsewhere in the gut, can be manifest in the mouth.

CHEILITIS/ANGULAR STOMATITIS
Inflammation of the corner of the mouth (**9**) can be due to a number of causes. Chronic candidal infection is frequent in edentulous patients; streptococcal and staphylococcal infections are more common in those with teeth. Riboflavin deficiency (vitamin B_2) causes a smooth 'magenta' tongue, angular stomatitis and, eventually, paraesthesia, photophobia, and blurred vision.

GEOGRAPHIC TONGUE
This is an oval or 'map'-shaped area on the dorsum of the tongue, with a well-defined margin and no known cause. It is asymptomatic, although some patients complain of sensitivity to spicy foods. Patients should be reassured.

GLOSSITIS
A red painful tongue can be caused by candidal infection and by deficiency of iron, vitamin B_{12}, folate, or riboflavin ('magenta tongue') (**10**).

APHTHOUS ULCERS
Mouth ulcers (**11**) can be intensely painful lesions.

Epidemiology and aetiology
About 20% of the population suffers from mouth ulcers, and the point prevalence is 2%. The condition is most present in the first two decades of life. Females are slightly more frequently affected than males. One-third of patients recognize foods as triggering attacks. Cessation of smoking may also provoke episodes.

Special forms
Minor aphthae
These are the most common form of lesions, appearing every couple of months in crops. They are 1–10 mm, round or ovoid with a 'punched-out' appearance, and affect only the gingival and hard palate – the nonkeratinized epithelium. The lesions heal after 3–14 days, usually without scarring.

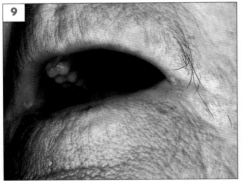

9 Cheilitis: painful areas at the corner of the mouth, in a patient with chronic iron deficiency.

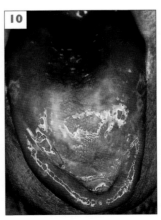

10 A smooth, painful tongue caused by vitamin B_2 deficiency.

Major aphthae
The lesions are larger than minor aphthae and can last longer – up to several months, sometimes scarring.

Herpetiform aphthae
These are named after their resemblance to herpetic lesions. They occur in crops of up to 100 small, 2–3 mm lesions, which are scattered throughout the mouth.

Differential diagnosis
A number of gastrointestinal diseases can manifest as recurrent oral ulceration. These include Crohn's disease, coeliac disease, Behçet's disease, and, less floridly, ulcerative colitis.

Laboratory and special examinations
Deficiency of iron, folate, and vitamin B_{12} must be excluded.

Pathophysiology
The cause of mouth ulcers is unknown. There is speculation regarding viral initiation, or an autoimmune reaction based on crossreactivity between food and bacterial antigens. A weak association with HLA-A2 is reported. The inflammatory infiltrate is lymphocytic and monocytic.

Prognosis
Crops of minor aphthae can recur for years; major aphthae may be more frequent and persist for longer. Episodes of herpetiform aphthae desist after a few years.

Management options
Acute episodes are treated with tetracycline mouthwashes, topical anaesthetic lozenges, and topical anti-inflammatory agents to relieve the pain. Corticosteroids can be given as pastes or pellets, or rarely systemically for severe disease. Thalidomide has been used in refractory ulcers associated with human immunodeficiency virus (HIV) and Behçet's disease.

Nutritional deficiency should be sought and corrected. Progesterone may benefit the minority of women with menstrual-related symptoms.

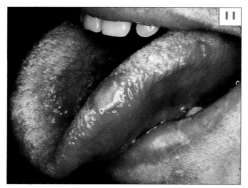

11 Aphthous ulcer – suggesting inflammation in the bowel (Crohn's disease, coeliac disease).

Oral cancer

History
Patients complain of an enlarging lump or ulcer. Lesions may bleed and are initially painless.

Physical examination
Exophytic and ulcerating lesions are seen. Although these lesions can arise anywhere in the mouth and pharynx, 50% involve the lips or tongue. Multiple lesions are not uncommon.

Epidemiology and aetiology
The disease is more common in men than in woman, and the average age at presentation is 60 years. The major causative factors are smoking, chewing tobacco, and drinking alcohol. Other factors include chronic irritation from ill-fitting dentures, and chronic infections such as *Candida* and syphilis (**12**). Leukoplakia and, in the Far East, submucous fibrosis (associated with chewing tobacco, betel, and eating chillies) are premalignant conditions.

Differential diagnosis
Other causes of oral ulceration have no specific features, so all oral ulcers of more than 2 weeks' duration must be biopsied. An indurated ulcer base and hard everted edges are suggestive of carcinoma.

Laboratory and special examinations
Histological assessment is mandatory.

Pathophysiology
About 90% of lesions are squamous cell carcinomas, which spread by local invasion. Distant metastases are rare.

Prognosis
The prognosis for oral cancer is poor.

Management options
Alcohol and tobacco must be discontinued, as there is a 20% chance of a secondary head and neck cancer. En-bloc resection and radiotherapy offer the best chance of prolonged survival.

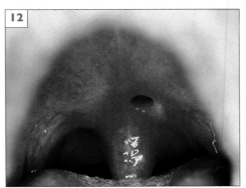

12 A perforated hard palate – the gumma of tertiary syphilis.

Oral keratoses and leukoplakia

KERATOSES

Excessive keratinization of the oral mucosa presents as a white patch. It occurs in a number of conditions, including:

- Chronic irritation (smoking, poorly fitting dentures).
- Idiopathic leukoplakia.
- Lichen planus.
- Lupus erythematosus.
- *Candida* infection.
- Hairy leukoplakia (an Epstein–Barr virus associated lesion, mostly confined to patients infected with HIV).

If white lesions cannot be scraped off (as for instance with *Candida* pseudomembranes) and other causes are excluded, it is termed leukoplakia.

LEUKOPLAKIA

This is a premalignant lesion, with up to 5% progress to cancer – especially lesions on the floor of the mouth and in those with erythema. Biopsy is mandatory; thermal surgery and topical cytotoxic therapy are the management options.

LICHEN PLANUS

This is a benign lesion, the most common intraoral keratosis, which can manifest anywhere in the mouth or on the tongue.

History

Oral lesions are usually asymptomatic and found incidentally, often during dental examination (in contrast to skin lesions, which are pruritic).

Physical examination

For reticular or papular lesions, Wickham's striae – forming a reticulated, fine lacy white pattern over the lesions – are characteristic. Concurrent cutaneous lesions are violaceous, with a polygonal planar lesion found particularly on the flexor aspect of the wrists and ankles.

Epidemiology and aetiology

Lichen planus occurs after the third decade.

Special forms

- Hypertrophic: often asymptomatic.
- Erosive: large shallow painful ulcers, which can be complicated by infection.
- Bullous: rare. If bullae burst, they form ulcers.

Differential diagnosis

Local lichenified eruptions are associated with drugs, and some dental amalgams. Leukoplakia and erythroplakia are present.

Laboratory and special examinations

Histology shows hyperkeratosis, hyperplasia, and liquefaction of the basal cell layer. There is dense lymphocytic infiltration of the dermoepidermal junction.

Pathophysiology

Unknown. The condition may be precipitated by drugs (nonsteroidal anti-inflammatory drugs (NSAIDs), sulphasalazine). There is a possible association with hepatitis C infection.

Prognosis

Unlike the cutaneous disease, which resolves after 18–24 months, oral lichen planus is more persistent. Atrophic and erosive causes may progress to malignancy in about 2% of cases.

Management options

Withdrawal of precipitating drugs, if this is the suspected cause.

Bullous lesions

PEMPHIGUS VULGARIS

This is a rare disease, which affects both sexes equally. Oral involvement occurs in 50% of patients. Fluid-filled bullae burst, to leave painful shallow ulcers that resolve over weeks or months. The disease is relapsing and remitting. Antibodies to intraepithelial antigens can be detected. The key histological feature is acantholytic cells, and the bullae form from suprabasal layers. Treatment by systemic steroids, with or without azathioprine, is required indefinitely.

PEMPHIGOID

Pemphigoid is another rare skin disorder producing bullous lesions in the mouth. It is more common in men and affects an older age group than pemphigus vulgaris. Subepithelial bullae form as the epithelium detaches from the lamina propria; the bullae then rupture to leave ulcers. The condition may involve the mouth, other mucous membranes, or the eye.

In addition to steroids, dapsone may be helpful in treatment.

ERYTHEMA MULTIFORME

This occurs at all ages, and is more common in men. In its severest form, it produces painful mucosal erosions and ulcers in the oral cavity. Oral involvement can occur in the absence of skin lesions, making the diagnosis difficult, and it must be differentiated from other bullous diseases.

Management consists of withdrawing the precipitating drug if it can be identified.

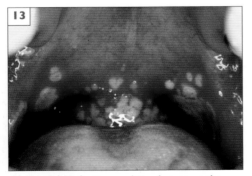

13 Candidal infection – white plaques on the palate.

Treatment is by tetracycline mouthwashes and steroids.

HERPETIC GINGIVITIS

Herpetic gingivitis occurs in young children. There may be systemic illness with fever, sore throat, and lymphadenopathy, followed by vesicle formation throughout the mouth. The vesicles ulcerate, coalesce, and form large confluent areas of shallow ulceration.

Treatment is symptomatic: tetracycline mouthwashes to hinder secondary bacterial infection, and aciclovir for severe disease.

INFECTIVE GINGIVITIS (SYNONYM VINCENT'S INFECTION)

Bacterial infection of the gingival membrane can produce haemorrhagic gingival ulceration. This may affect all ages, and is more common in smokers. Mixed organisms – largely mouth flora – are responsible, including Gram-negative anaerobes. Poor dental hygiene is important in the aetiopathogenesis. Severe disease occurs in immunocompromised patients. Patients complain of pain, bleeding gums, halitosis, regional lymphadenopathy, and sometimes fever.

Prevention involves careful oral toilet in debilitated and acutely ill patients at risk of infection. Antibiotics, dental cleaning, and mouthwashes are used to treat established infection.

CANDIDA (SYNONYM THRUSH)

Candida is a common oral commensal, but infection is unusual in the absence of predisposing factors such as antibiotics, systemic illness, immunosuppression, and xerostomia (dry mouth, as in Sjögren's syndrome). White plaques are the most common manifestation (**13**), but painful glossitis and cheilitis are also seen. Palatal *Candida* can present as a painful erythematous plaque in edentulous patients, sometimes in association with cheilitis.

A chronic hyperplastic form of *Candida*, with firm diffuse plaques, affects patients with acute immunodeficiency syndrome (AIDS) as part of chronic mucocutaneous candidiasis.

Treatment with oral antifungals is sufficient for most patients, but systemic treatment is indicated for chronic mucocutaneous candidiasis.

Oesophagus

Dysphagia is a potentially sinister symptom that requires investigation

Endoscopy is the most valuable form of investigation, but both barium radiology and motility studies may be helpful

Heartburn (pyrosis) due to reflux is common and may lead to oesophagitis. The relationship between hiatus hernia and reflux has been overemphasized in the past

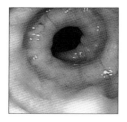
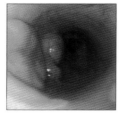
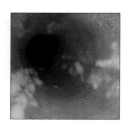
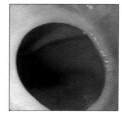

Anatomy/histology

The oesophagus is a muscular tube, which runs from the cricopharyngeal to the oesophagogastric junction. Anatomically, in the normal adult, the oesophagogastric junction is approximately 38 cm from the incisor teeth.

Histologically, the mucosal lining comprises squamous epithelium, with surrounding layers of circular and longitudinal muscle. There are normal regenerative 'pegs' in the epithelium.

Investigating the oesophagus

Endoscopy and barium radiology represent the primary means by which structural diseases of the oesophagus may be investigated. Newer developments in wireless capsule endoscopy may change this – see Chapter 5.

RADIOLOGY

The classical radiological investigation of the oesophagus has been the barium swallow (**14**). Structural lesions, such as ulcers and strictures, are readily identified (**15**), and the technique is more sensitive than endoscopy in detecting extrinsic compression of the oesophagus. It is better and safer than endoscopy for the examination of oesophageal pouches, webs, and rings, since it is performed without sedation or instrumentation.

A plain chest X-ray may occasionally be helpful, revealing either the position of swallowed foreign bodies (**16**), or demonstrating gross dilatation of the oesophagus, as in achalasia.

Mucosal disease

Barium radiology is less sensitive than endoscopy for small mucosal lesions, and cannot reliably differentiate benign from malignant strictures. These should be assessed by endoscopic biopsy. Barium swallow should precede endoscopy in the investigation of 'high' dysphagia. The endoscopist is forewarned, to prevent the rare but potentially dangerous situation of intubating a pharyngeal pouch (potentially leading to perforation). Endoscopic biopsy also indicates the level and likely nature of an obstructing lesion.

14 Normal barium swallow appearances.

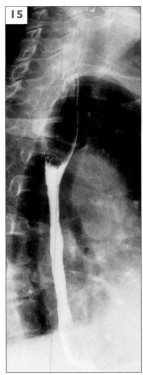

15 A long stricture in the oesophagus due to ingestion of caustic soda.

Reflux
Reflux of barium from the stomach into the oesophagus can be demonstrated. However, since this can be provoked in many normal subjects, it is not a reliable discriminator.

Motility
Swallowing disorders can be investigated using videofluoroscopy. Although the technique can also detect gross motility disorders affecting the body of the oesophagus, such as advanced achalasia or diffuse oesophageal spasm, manometry is more sensitive.

ENDOSCOPY
Upper gastrointestinal endoscopy is now routine, and the key investigation in upper gastrointestinal symptomatology (**17**). The low risk of complications is primarily related to the sedation that most patients are given, and to perforation and haemorrhage following instrumentation. The immediate advantage of endoscopy over barium radiology is the ability to take samples for histological and cytological assessment. This is mandatory in the assessment of oesophageal ulcers and strictures.

Reflux
Mucosal changes (ranging from subtle reddening to mucosal ulceration) can be detected in patients with gastro-oesophageal reflux disease. However, in 30% of cases, the endoscopic and histological appearances remain normal.

Motility
Although endoscopy is of no value in the diagnosis of motility disorders *per se*, patients with achalasia require endoscopy to exclude malignancy at the lower oesophagus or gastric cardia. Conversely, oesophageal motility disorders may be secondary to oesophagitis.

ENDOSCOPIC ULTRASOUND
High-resolution images of the oesophageal wall and adjacent structures can be obtained using endoscopic ultrasound (EUS), because the probe can be applied close to the lesion. Interfaces between layers in the gut wall are displayed as

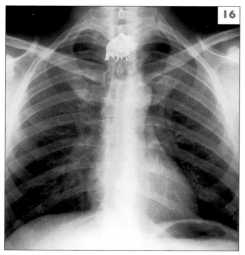

16 A foreign body (dental plate) lodged in the oesophagus.

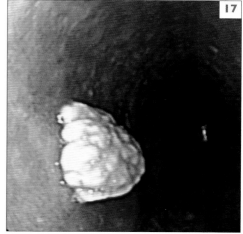

17 An incidental finding of a benign oesophageal lesion — a papilloma seen and biopsied at endoscopy.

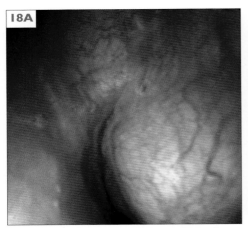

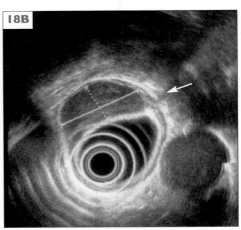

18 A submucosal lesion in the oesophagus. Seen at endoscopy (**A**), it appears as a smooth bulge and it is impossible to determine if this is extrinsic to the oesophagus. Using EUS (**B**), a gastrointestinal tumour is clearly seen as arising from the intrinsic layers of the oesophagus.

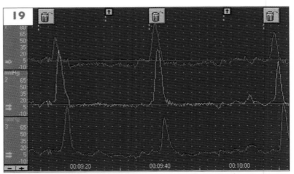

19 Oesophageal manometry. Normal study showing the wave of peristalsis progressing down the oesophagus.

concentric rings. The technique has proved valuable in assessing local spread of oesophageal tumours, and permits guided fine needle aspiration or biopsy of mediastinal structures (e.g. lymph nodes, 18).

OESOPHAGEAL PH STUDIES
Oesophageal pH monitoring detects reflux of acid into the oesophagus by use of a pH meter probe on a fine tube. The technique is unnecessary in most patients with gastro-oesophageal reflux disease, and is reserved for patients with an atypical history and those presenting with obscure chest pain. The frequency and duration of episodes of oesophageal reflux can be investigated by placing a pH electrode above the lower oesophageal sphincter. The gold standard is the percentage of time the intraoesophageal pH is <4 during a 24-hr period. This varies with age, but a value of >7% is abnormal in young people.

The sensitivity of the distal oesophagus to acid can be formally assessed by the Bernstein acid perfusion test, but this is now rarely performed.

MANOMETRY

Cine- or videofluoroscopy is used to assess oropharyngeal disorders where a food bolus cannot transit to the oesophagus. However, motility disorders of the body of the oesophagus are best investigated by manometry. An oesophageal catheter records pressure at multiple levels in the oesophagus. The pressure records of spontaneous and swallowing-induced motor activity are recorded and analysed (**19**). Indications for oesophageal manometry include unexplained dysphagia, chest pain, and the presurgical evaluation of patients with reflux.

OESOPHAGEAL SCINTIGRAPHY

Oesophageal function can also be investigated using oesophageal scintigraphy, although this is now rare in clinical practice. Patients swallow a standard meal or drink containing a nonabsorbable radiolabelled tracer, which is detected by a gamma-camera. Motility disorders are detected by measuring the scintigraphic oesophageal transit, and scintigraphic tests of reflux generally correlate with oesophageal pH tests. Although now rarely used, oesophageal scintigraphy is quick, noninvasive, and repeatable. In addition, as the radiation dose is less than conventional radiology, the technique is useful in longitudinal studies and paediatric patients.

Benign oesophageal tumours

Benign oesophageal tumours are reported during upper gastrointestinal endoscopy, either as an incidental finding or in patients with symptoms of dysphagia. They arise from any of the mucosal layers – at endoscopy submucosal lesions are covered by normal mucosa and appear as smooth indentations (e.g. lipomas).

MANAGEMENT

In practice, the key issue is differentiation from a malignant lesion. Biopsy of mucosal lesions at endoscopy is usually diagnostic – polypoid lesions can be snared endoscopically (**17**). EUS with aspiration biopsy is useful in determining from which layer the lesion arises, and will facilitate diagnosis of leiomyomas (the commonest intramucosal lesion, **18**). Surgical resection is required for large lesions and when the diagnosis remains uncertain.

Carcinoma of the oesophagus

Definition

Carcinoma of the oesophagus is defined as primary cancer of the oesophagus. Squamous cell carcinoma and adenocarcinoma account for more than 90% of cases.

Epidemiology and aetiology

Carcinoma of the oesophagus primarily affects those aged over 65 years, and is more common in men than women. In the West, there has been an alarming increase in oesophageal adenocarcinoma during recent decades, while squamous cell carcinoma of the oesophagus has declined. There are interesting geographic variations in disease incidence, suggesting that environmental factors are important in aetiology. Iran, China, and parts of southern Africa have the highest rates. For squamous cell carcinoma, alcohol and tobacco use are independent aetiological factors, which also act synergistically. Dietary factors include deficiency of trace elements and vitamins, intake of nitrites and nitrosamines, and (in China) fungal contamination of foods. For oesophageal adenocarcinoma, the predisposing factors include Barrett's oesophagus and, possibly, gastro-oesophageal reflux *per se*, chronic oesophagitis, peptic oesophageal ulceration, and leukoplakia.

Pathophysiology

The macroscopic appearances range from ulcer, to exophytic lesions and strictures. Squamous cell carcinoma is most common in the upper third of the oesophagus. Such carcinomas are generally radiosensitive and have a better prognosis than adenocarcinomas, which are more frequent in the distal oesophagus. Adenocarcinomas arise in the columnar-lined mucosa of Barrett's oesophagus. The disease spreads locally, circumferentially in submucosal tissue, and into the adjacent mediastinal structures, including the trachea, pericardium, and aorta. Lymphatic spread is common.

Clinical history

Dysphagia is the dominant symptom. Usually, this is relentlessly progressive, but in some patients the first manifestation of disease is complete dysphagia from an obstructing bolus of food. Regurgitation eventually occurs. Other symptoms may include pain on swallowing and cough. Cough may represent aspiration, or the development of an oesophagotracheal fistula. Recurrent laryngeal nerve palsy, due to mediastinal spread, causes hoarseness.

Physical examination

Examination is abnormal only in advanced disease. Secondary deposits may be palpable in supraclavicular lymph nodes. Mediastinal spread may lead to superior vena cava obstruction.

Laboratory and special investigations
Diagnosis

A barium swallow is sometimes the first investigation of dysphagia, and will demonstrate oesophageal cancer (**20**). However, endoscopic biopsy and brushing of any suspicious lesions is mandatory.

Staging

Prognosis and therapeutic approach are dictated by tumour staging, particularly in selecting the patients amenable to surgery. Computed tomography (CT) scanning will detect distant metastatic disease. In appropriate patients, local spread is assessed by EUS (**21**), to determine the depth of tumour invasion, and involvement of local lymph nodes and adjacent structures. Staging laparoscopy is indicated for distal oesophageal tumours. Additional assessments include positron-emission tomography (PET) using ^{18}F flourodeoxyglucose, which is more sensitive for metastatic disease than CT (**22**). Cardiorespiratory assessment is indicated in those being considered for surgery.

Differential diagnosis

Gastric carcinoma spreading to the lower oesophagus may mimic oesophageal carcinoma. Lesions at the cardia may be misdiagnosed as achalasia when there is associated oesophageal dilatation (**23**). Peptic strictures may be indistinguishable from malignant strictures. Apparently benign 'peptic' strictures recurring soon after dilatation should be regarded with suspicion. A long history of reflux before the onset of dysphagia suggests benign peptic stricture, but biopsy remains mandatory.

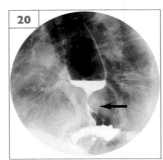

20 Barium swallow showing obstruction due to carcinoma of the oesophagus.

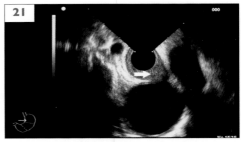

21 EUS. This is a radial image and shows eccentric thickening of the oesophageal wall due to a tumour (marked with arrow).

Special forms
Patterson–Kelly syndrome
(Plummer–Vinson syndrome)

In some women with long-standing iron-deficiency anaemia, chronic inflammatory changes associated with hyperkeratinization occur in the hypopharynx. Cricopharyngeal spasm causes dysphagia. This syndrome is generally benign, but may be complicated by squamous carcinoma.

Prognosis

The prognosis for oesophageal cancer is appalling, since more than 50% of patients present with advanced disease, and most of these patients are dead within a year of diagnosis.

Management
Curative

Surgery offers the best prospect of cure for adenocarcinoma. Preoperative platinum-based chemotherapy has been shown to improve

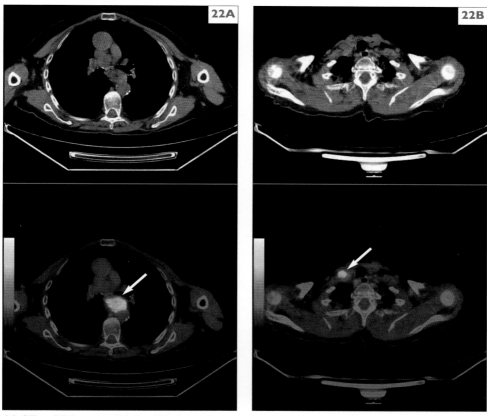

22 CT – PET images: (**A**) the CT of the primary oesophageal tumour; (**B**) metastatic disease in the supraclavicular nodes. (The PET scan is coregistered with the CT images.)

23 Cancer at the gastro-oesophageal junction seen at endoscopy with the endoscope retroflexed.

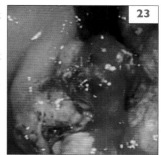

survival, compared to surgery alone. There is no evidence for postoperative chemoradiotherapy. The best results are obtained in patients with favourable tumours in the middle or lower third of the oesophagus, treated by partial oesophagectomy or oesophagogastrectomy, respectively. This is a disease of the elderly and has high operative mortality rates. Surgery is only appropriate in adequately nourished patients with sufficient cardiorespiratory reserve. Chemoradiotherapy is appropriate for tumours adjacent to other structures, which renders them unresectable. For squamous cell carcinoma of the upper and middle oesophagus, concurrent chemoradiotherapy may be as effective as surgery, based on indirect comparisons.

Palliative

Dysphagia is a distressing symptom for patients and their relatives, and is the principal symptom requiring palliation. Depending on the available expertise, a number of options can be tailored to the individual patient:

- Endoscopic dilatation of malignant strictures, which will temporarily palliate impending oesophageal obstruction.
- Direct endoscopic ablation therapy of the tumour using laser, argon-plasma coagulation, or injection of alcohol into the tumour.
- Oesophageal stent. As an alternative to endoscopic ablation, self-expanding metal oesophageal stents can be placed either endoscopically or using fluoroscopic guidance (24), to maintain oesophageal patency. The stents are made from memory metal and are delivered in a compact form. Once in the appropriate position, they are deployed and expand. Although simpler to place than the older rigid stents previously used, and well tolerated by patients, they are still subject to the potential complications of bleeding, stent migration, and oesophageal perforation. Subsequent tumour overgrowth of the stent can cause obstruction, which can usually be controlled by endoscopic means.

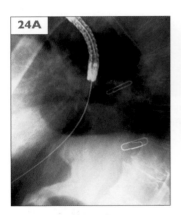

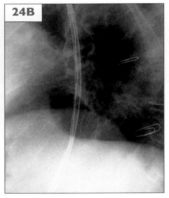

24 Palliation of oesophageal cancer with a self-expanding metal stent. This sequence shows placement of a guidewire across the cancer and then deployment of the stent.

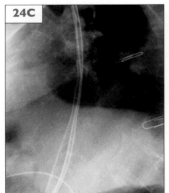

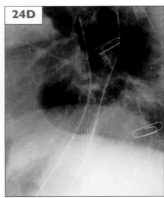

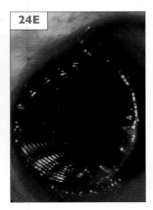

Achalasia and other primary motility disorders

The motility disorders of the oesophagus include inadequate lower oesophageal sphincter relaxation (typified by achalasia), uncoordinated contraction and hypercontraction (such as diffuse oesophageal spasm), and hypocontraction with ineffective oesophageal motility. In clinical practice, patients can show mixed abnormalities, and these categories are not absolute (**25**). Oesophageal dysmotility can arise as a primary disorder or reflect a systemic disease, as in scleroderma, for example (**26**).

Achalasia is a condition of unknown aetiology, associated with absent oesophageal peristalsis and failure of relaxation of the lower oesophageal sphincter (LOS).

Epidemiology and aetiology
Achalasia is rare and affects both sexes equally. It occurs in adults of any age.

Pathophysiology
The key feature is ganglion loss from the myenteric neural plexus, which can be demonstrated histologically and is supported by pharmacological evidence of denervation. Progressive oesophageal dilatation arises from a combination of lack of peristalsis and failure of relaxation of the LOS. Diffuse thickening of the wall occurs from secondary changes in mucosal and smooth muscle layers.

Clinical history
Dysphagia
This is progressive and – in contrast to most causes – characteristically presents with dysphagia for both liquids and solids from the outset.

Regurgitation
Postprandial regurgitation may be described as vomiting by the patient, but it is generally effortless, without retching. Regurgitation on recumbency can lead to aspiration and repeated chest infections. Younger patients may complain of retrosternal chest pain.

Physical examination
There may be no physical signs.

Laboratory and special examinations
Barium studies in achalasia are variable. The oesophagus may be dilated and tortuous with a fluid level (sometimes visible on a routine chest radiograph), and 'bird's beak' tapering at the lower oesophageal sphincter (**27**). No

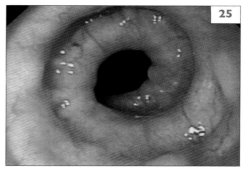

25 Endoscopic view of corkscrew oesophagus.

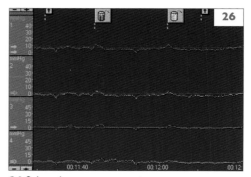

26 Scleroderma manometric trace.

27 Achalasia: barium swallow – note the characteristic dilated oesophagus with fluid level, with a 'bird's beak' tapering at the oesophago-gastric junction.

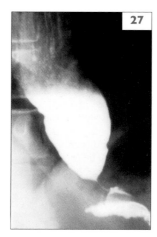

peristalsis is seen on screening, and in advanced cases the gastric air bubble is absent. In manometric studies, resting lower oesophageal sphincter pressures may be elevated and relaxation is absent. Simultaneous pressure peaks (i.e. no propulsive contractions) are seen in the oesophageal body on swallowing (**28**).

Special forms
Megaoesophagus associated with absent peristalsis occurs in amyloid. Paraneoplastic manifestations of carcinoma of the pancreas, stomach, and bronchus may mimic achalasia, but these patients have a shorter history of dysphagia (<1 year), and disproportionate weight loss. Secondary forms are seen in diabetic or alcoholic neuropathy, pseudo-obstruction, and Chagas' disease (parasitic infection due to *Trypanosoma cruzi*).

Differential diagnosis
Carcinoma of the gastric cardia may both mimic and complicate achalasia. Endoscopy and biopsy are therefore mandatory. Endoscopy is a frequent investigation in patients with dysphagia; although achalasia cannot be diagnosed in this way, it may be suspected when undigested food debris is seen in the oesophagus.

Prognosis
Squamous carcinoma may arise in the dilated segment. Respiratory complications may arise from aspiration.

Management
Medical therapy is unsatisfactory, although reduction in lower oesophageal sphincter pressure may be attempted with isosorbide dinitrate or calcium antagonists. Endoscopic treatment using botulinum toxin injection into the lower oesophageal sphincter, to inhibit cholinergic neurones and facilitate sphincter relaxation, has been described as both a diagnostic and therapeutic approach. Better (and longer-term) symptom control is achieved by disrupting the circular muscle fibres – either endoscopic pneumatic dilatation or surgical myotomy using a modified Heller's procedure (longitudinal slit through oesophageal muscle or cardia).

Abnormal peristalsis in the absence of mucosal lesion is seen in other conditions, as well as in achalasia.

DIFFUSE OESOPHAGEAL SPASM
Epidemiology and aetiology
This is rare, but occurs in patients aged over 50 years, and in both sexes.

Pathophysiology
The pathophysiology of diffuse oesophageal spasm is not known.

Clinical history
Patients complain principally of retrosternal chest pain, with the character and distribution of angina. In 50% of patients, episodes are precipitated by eating but may also occur nocturnally. Symptoms may deteriorate under emotional stress. Some patients also have dysphagia.

Physical examination
Physical examination is normal.

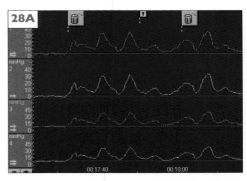

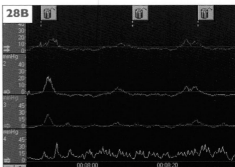

28 Achalasia: the manometric trace is usually characterized by no peristaltic waves, incomplete or absent oesophageal sphincter relaxation, and commonly, a raised basal lower oesophageal sphincter pressure.

Laboratory and special examinations

Manometric abnormalities are similar to achalasia, but are less marked. Simultaneous, repetitive, high-amplitude 'tertiary' contractions are seen in the middle third of the oesophagus (29, 30). A variety of segmental, nonperistaltic contractions are seen on barium examination. Oesophageal dilatation and retained food debris are unusual.

Other forms

Hypertensive lower oesophageal sphincter syndrome

Patients have elevated resting lower oesophageal sphincter tone, occurring alone or in association with nutcracker oesophagus (**31**) – which describes abnormally high distal oesophageal contractions, presenting with angina-like chest pain.

Irritable oesophagus

Patients have symptoms of noncardiac chest pain, caused at different times by either acid reflux or dysmotility. Irritable oesophagus can be identified by 24-hr intraoesophageal pH and pressure measurements.

Differential diagnosis

Angina presents with a similar pain. In patients with achalasia, dysphagia is the predominant symptom.

Prognosis and treatment

Sublingual glyceryl trinitrate will relieve the pain of oesophageal spasm. Myotomy or dilatation is rarely indicated. Management of irritable oesophagus is generally unsatisfactory, and treatment must be directed towards either dysmotility or reflux as appropriate.

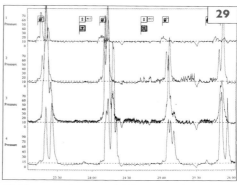

29 Maonmetric trace of diffuse oesophageal spasm (DOS).

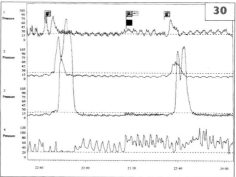

30 Nutcracker oesophagus: manometric trace – high-pressure contractions of extended duration.

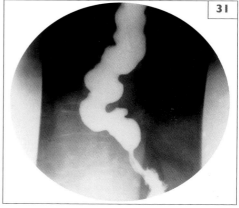

31 Nutcracker oesophagus; barium swallow – note irregular, nonpropulsive, incoordinate contraction of the oesophagus.

Gastro-oesophageal reflux disease and oesophagitis

Definition
The terminology of gastro-oesophageal reflux disease and oesophagitis is confused. Reflux of gastric contents is a normal occurrence postprandially, and is only considered abnormal if it gives rise to symptoms – referred to as gastro-oesophageal reflux disease (GORD).

Oesophagitis refers to the subsequent oesophageal mucosal injury that occurs in a minority of patients (**32**).

Epidemiology and aetiology
Up to one-third of the population have symptoms of reflux, but oesophagitis occurs in only a minority of these. Apart from during pregnancy, when it is a common complaint, symptoms are more severe in those aged over 50 years – possibly reflecting an age-related decline in oesophageal motor function. Smoking and obesity are aggravating factors, while NSAIDs (including aspirin) are definite aetiological factors, and may act by reducing mucosal defence against injury.

Helicobacter pylori infection does not seem to play a significant role.

Pathophysiology
The intraoesophageal pH is <4 for a greater percentage of the time in patients compared with controls, and this is correlated with the degree of mucosal injury. Two abnormalities are commonly detected in patients:
- Gastric juice refluxes into the oesophagus during episodes when lower oesophageal sphincter tone is transiently reduced.
- Oesophageal clearance of the refluxate is impaired.

There is controversy as to the importance of sliding hiatus hernia in the pathogenesis of GORD. Movement of the lower oesophageal sphincter to the thorax from the abdomen means that it is subject to negative intrathoracic pressures, and therefore loses the protective effect of coordinated contractions of the diaphragmatic crurae. These abnormalities increase the likelihood of reflux episodes on straining. The quality of the refluxate is rarely important, unless the patient has Zollinger–Ellison syndrome (gross gastric hyperacidity stimulated by a

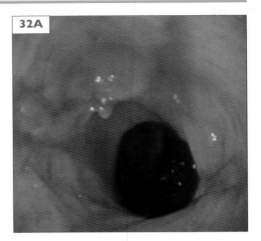

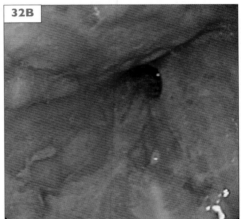

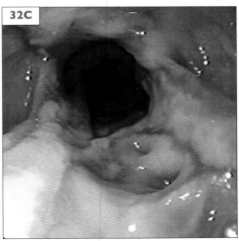

32 Various degrees of reflux oesophagitis, with ulceration through to scarring and puckering.

neuroendocrine tumour releasing the hormone gastrin). Bile is an irritant and increases oesophageal injury. However, except after gastric surgery, biliary reflux is uncommon.

The histological changes in the mucosa range from mild inflammation, to complete denuding of the squamous epithelium.

Clinical history

The most distinctive symptom is heartburn. Typically, it is experienced postprandially and is exacerbated by large, fatty meals. Some patients associate symptoms with particular foods. Bloating, nausea, anorexia, regurgitation, and odynophagia also occur.

Dysphagia occurs either as a consequence of a secondary motility disorder or, less commonly, because of a peptic stricture (**33**). Respiratory symptoms arising from oesophagopharyngeal reflux are rare, but may underlie some cases of asthma. Pharyngeal symptoms and symptoms of heartburn are not reported in a substantial proportion of patients.

Physical examination

There are no physical signs.

Laboratory and special investigations

In a young patient with typical symptoms, investigation is unnecessary. The mucosal damage is usually confined to the distal 5 cm of the oesophagus, and is best assessed at endoscopy.

Oesophagitis can be graded, lesions brushed and biopsied, and the presence of columnar-lined oesophagus determined.

Oesophageal pH monitoring (**34**) is reserved for the patient with atypical symptoms or obscure chest pains, and for the investigation of reflux in relationship to respiratory symptoms.

Differential diagnosis

The diagnosis is usually straightforward. Other causes of distal oesophageal ulceration include CMV, herpes, and *Candida* in the immunocompromised.

Strictures associated with oesophagitis need to be differentiated from malignant strictures.

Prognosis

For most patients, GORD is a chronic condition with intermittent exacerbations of symptoms. Patients with severe circumferential oesophagitis are at risk of peptic stricture and columnar-lined oesophagus.

Management

The aim of treatment is symptomatic relief and the prevention of complications. This requires a graded approach. Patients with minimal symptoms and no mucosal damage should be treated conservatively, by avoiding precipitating factors, and should lose weight. Preventing reflux at night by elevating the head of the bed may help.

Pharmacological

Acid suppression with proton pump inhibitors or H_2 receptor antagonists is the mainstay of treatment. A step-down approach has been advocated – starting with high-dose acid suppression with proton pump inhibitor therapy and stepping down to a reduced dose or H_2 receptor antagonist. However, many patients will not achieve adequate symptom relief without proton pump inhibitors.

Endoscopic and surgical approaches

Antireflux surgery is an option for patients with refractory symptoms, stricture, haemorrhage (rare), or respiratory complications. The traditional fundoplication operation can be undertaken laparoscopically. Various endoscopic treatments of GORD have recently been advocated. These include, among others, an

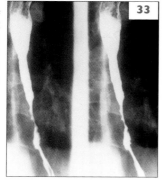

33 Extensive reflux oesophageal stricture seen on barium study.

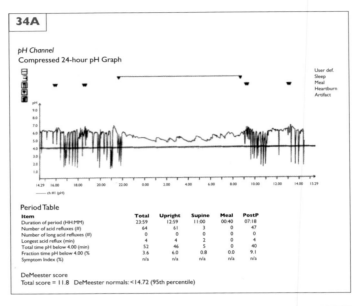

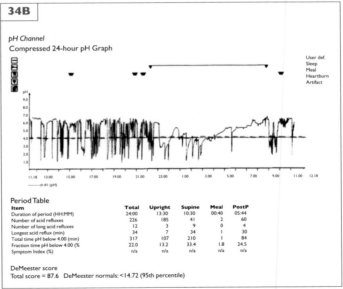

34 24-hr oesophageal pH monitoring, showing frequent episodes of reflux (low pH): (A) normal, (B) severe.

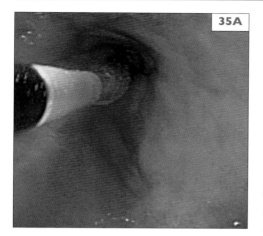

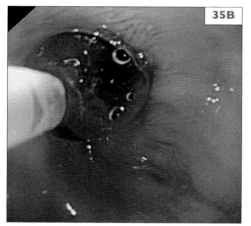

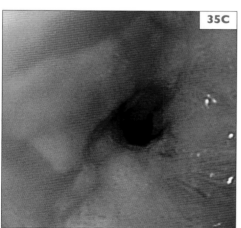

35 Endoscopic series of balloon dilatation of peptic stricture of oesophagus.

endoscopically placed plication to reduce reflux, or a submucosal injection of polymer at the gastro-oesophageal junction.

Complications

Peptic strictures can be dilated either endoscopically or by using a balloon under radiographic control if symptomatic dysphagia occurs (**35**).

Common causes of oesophagitis

The most common form of oesophagitis is peptic oesophagitis, caused by gastro-oesophageal reflux. The other main causes are pill oesophagitis and caustic oesophagitis.

Pill oesophagitis

Pill oesophagitis is characterized by acute oesophageal mucosal inflammation, caused by ingestion of medication. A number of drugs have been implicated, including tetracyclines, potassium supplements, certain bisphosphonates, and some NSAIDs. The presentation is with dysphagia, chest pain, or odynophagia, following ingestion of the medication. Stopping the causative pill, together with acid suppression therapy, is the usual approach. Patients are advised to remain upright for 30 minutes after such taking medications, and to accompany the tablets with plenty of fluid.

Caustic oesophagitis

Ingestion of caustic chemicals induces a rapid, dramatic, and sometimes fatal oesophagitis. Long-term sequelae include strictures and carcinoma (**15**).

Eosinophilic oesophagitis

Epidemiology and aetiology
Eosinophilic oesophagitis is being increasingly diagnosed, although it is still an unusual condition. This might be ascertainment bias, with increased recognition of the condition. Males are more frequently diagnosed.

Pathophysiology
Eosinophils are uncommon in the healthy oesophagus. The pathological hallmark of eosinophilic oesophagitis is eosinophilic infiltration of the mucosa; more than 20 per high-power field, with lesser degrees seen in GORD (**36**). An associated eosinophilia in the peripheral blood is found in a proportion, as are raised serum IgE levels. This, and the frequent atopic history, has been interpreted as suggesting an allergic aetiology.

Clinical features
Patients frequently present with dysphagia or recurrent food bolus obstruction. At endoscopy, a number of appearances have been described, none of which are specific. Mucosal changes include furrows, corrugations, and vertical lines (**37**). The lumen may have a small calibre (**38**).

Management
Any GORD should be treated. Endoscopic dilatation should be considered for small-calibre oesophagus, but is associated with a higher rate of oesophageal perforation than peptic disease. Bolus obstruction can be managed endoscopically. There is no routine medical therapy, but topical steroids (fluticasone) and the leukotriene receptor antagonist montelukast have been used.

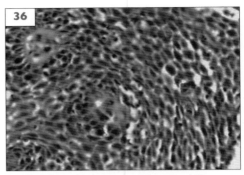

36 Histological appearance of eosinophilic oesophagitis.

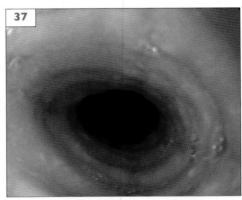

37 Eosinophilic oesophagitis – note vertical furrows.

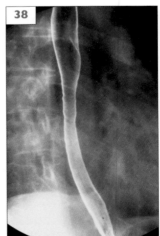

38 Barium swallow showing small-calibre oesophagus in a patient with long-standing eosinophilic oesophagitis.

Oesophageal varices

Definition
Oesophageal varices are defined as dilated intramural oesophageal veins. They are portosystemic venous communications, and the direct result of portal hypertension. Oesophageal varices can bleed, which makes them the most important manifestation of portal hypertension in clinical practice (**39, 40**).

Pathophysiology
Normally, all the blood delivered to the liver by the portal venous system returns through the liver to the systemic circulation via the hepatic veins. With cirrhosis, and when the portal venous system is obstructed, this does not occur. Portal venous pressure rises and portovenous shunts open to enable venous blood to return to the systemic circulation via alternative routes.

Clinical history
The patient may have a prior history of bleeding oesophageal varices, and of underlying liver disease.

Physical examination
Physical signs of portal hypertension include splenomegaly, dilated abdominal veins (flow is away from the umbilicus), and rectal varices. Since the principal cause of portal hypertension is liver cirrhosis, evidence of this is generally present.

Laboratory and special investigations
Oesophageal varices can be identified at barium swallow, and can be accentuated by a reverse Valsalva manoeuvre (**41**). However, endoscopy is a much better technique for detection, allowing the size of the varices to be assessed and indicating the presence of red signs (suggesting imminent risk of bleeding).

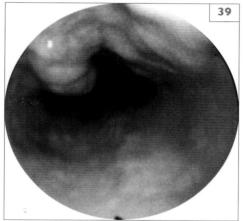

39 Oesophageal varices seen as varicose veins at endoscopy.

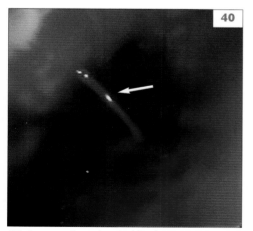

40 An oesophageal varix, bleeding.

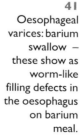

41 Oesophageal varices: barium swallow – these show as worm-like filling defects in the oesophagus on barium meal.

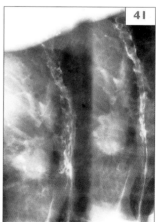

Other features of portal hypertension may be seen, e.g. gastric fundal varices (**42**) or portal hypertensive gastropathy. The latter has a range of endoscopic appearances, from a mosaic 'snakeskin' pattern, to a 'watermelon' stomach. Bleeding from portal hypertensive gastropathy is usually chronic and self-limiting, but patients can become anaemic.

The investigation of portal hypertension includes assessment of portal vein patency by Doppler ultrasound, or by CT or magnetic resonance (MR) angiography, and appropriate investigation of the liver. Portal pressures can be assessed indirectly by the difference between the wedged and free hepatic venous pressures, but this approach is not routine and is usually only carried out in specialized centres.

Special forms
Portal hypertension can occur in the absence of liver disease, for instance, portal vein thrombosis due to neonatal umbilical sepsis, instrumentation, or prothrombotic conditions. Splenic vein thrombosis also causes portal hypertension, especially gastric fundal varices, and is a complication of pancreatitis and blunt abdominal trauma (e.g. steering wheel injury in a road traffic accident). Other causes of noncirrhotic portal hypertension include congenital hepatic fibrosis and hepatic schistosomiasis. The importance of these uncommon conditions is that liver function is preserved, and the prognosis after variceal haemorrhage is much better.

Differential diagnosis
Gastrointestinal bleeding in patients who have oesophageal varices is not always variceal; peptic ulcers are more common in the cirrhotic population and these are said to be more difficult to heal. The gastric mucosa is also more sensitive to injury than normal.

Prognosis
Although only 30% of patients bleed from their oesophageal varices, the overall mortality rate for first bleed is around 50%. There are no reliable means of predicting which patients will bleed, but endoscopic signs are of some value. There is a greater risk of bleeding from larger varices (higher wall tension) and varices with 'red signs'. Bleeding risk is also higher in patients with more severe underlying liver disease and those with alcoholic liver disease.

Management
Prophylactic treatment
In alcoholic cirrhosis, abstinence will reduce the size of varices. Portal pressure can be reduced pharmacologically by propranolol or nadolol and, to a lesser extent, by oral nitrates, which can be tried in those intolerant of beta blockers. In order to reduce the risk of bleeding, the pressure gradient must be <12 mmHg. There is no place for prophylactic sclerotherapy, but prophylactic oesophageal band ligation can be pursued in patients with a high risk of bleeding, who are unsuitable for beta blocker therapy.

Bleeding
The management of bleeding oesophageal varices (discussed in Chapter 9) involves prompt resuscitation and haemodynamic monitoring. Variceal haemorrhage (**40**) is most effectively staunched by endoscopic therapy, either sclerotherapy, or more usually now, endoscopic variceal ligation (**43**). Balloon tamponade of bleeding varices is a temporizing measure, reserved for those who fail to respond to endoscopic therapy.

Drugs such as Glypressin or somatostatin cause acute reduction of portal pressure and blood flow, and should be considered as soon as possible.

The interventional radiological technique (TIPSS – transjugular intrahepatic portosystemic shunt) is reserved for patients who continue to bleed despite endoscopic and pharmacological therapy. A shunt is created from the hepatic vein to the portal vein, and a metal stent inserted. This prevents bleeding by directly lowering portal pressure. Direct surgical procedures of oversewing or ligating varices, or (less common nowadays) creation of a surgical shunt between portal and systemic vessels, can also be used in emergencies.

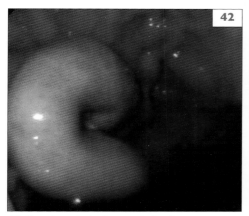

42 Gastric varix in the gastric fundus.

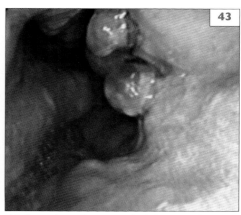

43 Oesophageal varices which have just been treated by 'banding'; that is, placing a rubber band about them.

Oesophageal webs and rings

Definition

Mucosal abnormalities are common in the oesophagus. Webs are folds of squamous mucosa that protrude into the lumen and may be found at all levels of the oesophagus. Rings are circumferential, with their upper surface covered by stratified squamous epithelium and columnar epithelium occurring on the lower surface.

The most commonly encountered type of mucosal abnormality is Schatzki's ring (**44, 45**), which occurs as a thin submucosal scar at the squamocolumnar junction.

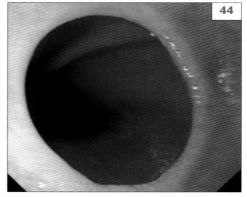

44 Oesophageal ring at endoscopy.

Aetiology and pathophysiology

It is proposed that Schatzki's rings arise in response to chronic injury by gastro-oesophageal reflux.

Clinical history

Some patients have no symptoms and the diagnosis is made incidentally. Dysphagia is unusual if the lumen is more than 20 mm. However, sudden complete dysphagia can occur due to obstruction of a bolus of food – the so-called 'steak-house syndrome'.

Management

Symptomatic rings or webs can be dilated and antireflux measures instituted.

45 Schatzki's ring – the faint indentation in the distal oesophagus seen on barium swallow.

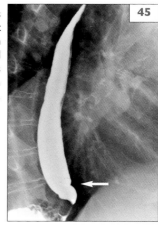

Oesophageal diverticula and pouches

Definition
Oesophageal diverticula are outpouchings of one or more layers of the oesophageal wall. They occur at three levels in the oesophagus – pharyngeal (immediately above the cricopharyngeus muscle), midoesophageal, and epiphrenic (just above the diaphragm).

Pharyngeal pouches
Also known as Zenker's diverticulum, these are the most important type, as they cause dysphagia and aspiration (**46–48**).

Midoesophageal diverticula
These are rarely symptomatic and arise either because of oesophageal dysmotility (pulsion) or because of mediastinal traction, e.g. from tuberculosis (**49**).

Epiphrenic diverticula
These occur in association with other diseases affecting oesophageal motility.

Aetiology, epidemiology, and pathophysiology
Pharyngeal pouches are uncommon and affect the elderly. The diverticula arise in the midline, posteriorly between the inferior constrictor and the cricopharyngeus muscles. They enlarge as thin-walled sacs, typically deviating to the left side of the neck. The aetiology may be failure of relaxation during swallowing, due to primary cricopharyngeal dysfunction, sometimes referred to as cricopharyngeal achalasia. There is an association with hiatus hernia.

Clinical history
Patients present variably with cough, dysphagia, regurgitation, and weight loss. There is a risk of aspiration.

Physical examination
Large pouches can sometimes be palpated in the neck after food has been eaten.

Laboratory and special examinations
Barium swallow is the most appropriate initial investigation (**47**). The pouch appears as a 'teapot spout'. Cine-radiology is helpful in early cases. Endoscopy should be performed cautiously, as the cricopharyngeal area is often a 'blind' region during intubation and this can be dangerous.

Prognosis
Complicating squamous carcinoma has been reported rarely.

Management
The standard approach is surgical. Options include cricopharyngeal myotomy, with or without excision of the pouch. Endoscopic stapling (Dohlman's procedure) is less invasive and patients – who are frequently elderly – may recover more quickly.

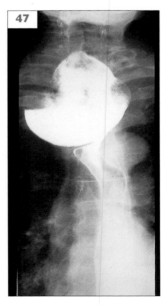

47 Barium swallow showing pharyngeal pouch.

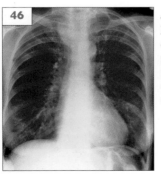

46 Chest X-ray showing outline of pharyngeal pouch in right upper mediastinum.

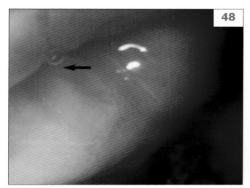

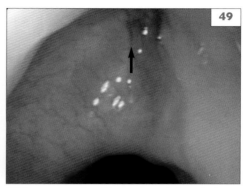

48 Endoscopic view of pharyngeal pouch. Note the entrance to the oesophagus in the upper left part of the picture, with food debris in the pouch to the bottom right of the picture. The natural path for the endoscope is into the pouch rather than the oesophagus.

49 Asymptomatic midoesophageal diverticulum at endoscopy.

Oesophageal infections

CANDIDAL OESOPHAGITIS

Candidal oesophagitis can be asymptomatic or can cause oesophageal pain, which is either persistent or occurs when swallowing (odynophagia). Like candidal infection elsewhere, it is more common in patients with diabetes, and in those receiving broad-spectrum antibiotic therapy or corticosteroid treatment. It also occurs under conditions of debilitation (including alcoholism) and immunosuppression (including AIDS, when pharyngeal plaques are sometimes seen (see **13**).

Examinations/investigations

Nodular plaques of *Candida* can be seen on barium swallow, or generalized ulceration may be visualized. At endoscopy, white plaques of *Candida* are seen on hyperaemic mucosa (**50**).

Differential diagnosis

Diagnosis can be confirmed from biopsies or brushings.

Management

Treatment is by antifungals, e.g. nystatin or amphotericin, given orally.

HERPETIC OESOPHAGITIS

Herpetic oesophagitis is most common in the immunocompromised, but has been reported in healthy people. It causes small vesicles and confluent superficial ulceration. Characteristic eosinophilic inclusions are seen on biopsy.

CYTOMEGALOVIRUS OESOPHAGITIS

Cytomegalovirus (CMV) is another cause of ulceration in the oesophagus and upper gastrointestinal tract of the immunocompromised. Immunohistochemical staining or an 'owl's eye' nuclear inclusion is diagnostic on histopathological examination.

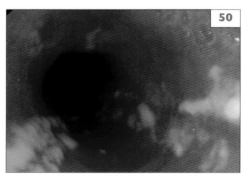

50 Oesophageal candidiasis: endoscopic appearance — fluffy white plaques of *Candida*.

Columnar-lined oesophagus (synonym Barrett's oesophagus)

Definition
Columnar-lined oesophagus is defined as the presence of columnar epithelium extending as a cylinder or tongues more than 3 cm up the oesophagus above the gastric cardia. The term short-segment Barrett's is reserved for cases where the metaplastic mucosa is shorter than the 3 cm used in the classical definition. Barrett's epithelium is similar to gastric lining epithelium and replaces the normal stratified squamous epithelium (**51**).

Epidemiology and aetiology
The average age at presentation is 55 years, and the disease is more common in Caucasian men. Columnar-lined oesophagus is found in up to 4% of patients at endoscopy, and in 20% of patients with oesophagitis.

Pathophysiology
The prevailing theory is that columnar-lined oesophagus is due to gastro-oesophageal reflux. Chronic oesophageal mucosal inflammation and desquamation of the squamous epithelium occurs in the distal oesophagus. This is replaced by columnar epithelium as an adaptive response, and thus the squamocolumnar junction migrates up the oesophagus. Gastro-oesophageal reflux is common in Barrett's patients, which supports this view.

Clinical history
Symptoms are usually due to the associated gastro-oesophageal reflux and oesophagitis.

Physical examination
There are no physical signs.

Laboratory and special examinations
The diagnosis is suspected at endoscopy. Normally, the demarcation between pink–grey squamous epithelium and salmon-red columnar epithelium forms an irregular ring at the cardia. This is called the ora serrata or 'Z' line. In columnar-lined oesophagus, this migrates proximally as a cylinder, with islands of pink squamous mucosa or long irregular tongues of columnar mucosa rising into the oesophagus from the cardia (**51**). Endoscopic mucosal biopsies must be taken at multiple sites, to confirm the gastric columnar epithelium and detect dysplasia. *Helicobacter pylori* infection of the gastric metaplasia may also be found.

Differential diagnosis
Columnar-lined oesophagus lacks the rugae of stomach mucosa, which distinguishes it from sliding hiatus herniae. In practice, a more

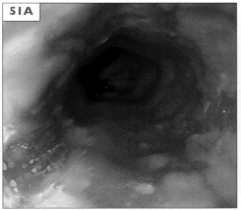
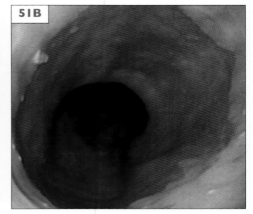

51 Two images of uncomplicated Barrett's oesophagus.

common error is for the endoscopist to overlook the diagnosis of Barrett's syndrome, since the colour change from the pink squamous mucosa to the salmon-red columnar epithelium can be subtle.

Prognosis

The importance of Barrett's oesophagus is that dysplasia and adenocarcinoma can arise in the specialized metaplastic mucosa (**52**). Estimates for the increased risk of developing adenocarcinoma range from 30 to 100 times that of age-matched controls.

Management

Gastro-oesophageal reflux and oesophagitis are treated conventionally. As yet, there is no firm evidence that proton pump inhibitors or surgery induce regression of the lesion, or reduce the risk of progression to adenocarcinoma.

Endoscopic surveillance

Regular endoscopic surveillance of patients with Barrett's oesophagus, with the aim of identifying dysplastic mucosa or early diagnosis of cancer, remains controversial. It is only worthwhile if the patient is prepared to accept oesophageal resection if high-grade dysplasia is detected. The economic benefit of surveillance is unclear. Current UK recommendations suggest 2-yearly quadratic biopsies of the Barrett's mucosa every 2 cm (with additional biopsies of any visible abnormalities).

Endoscopic surveillance of dysplasia

Following detection of low-grade dysplasia (and independent confirmation), the patient is re-evaluated after 8–12 weeks' intensive acid suppression. Patients with high-grade dysplasia should be considered for oesophagectomy, since the risk of coincident carcinoma is considerable.

Endoscopic treatment

Newer endoscopic treatments, to ablate columnar-lined oesophagus and 'resurface' with squamous mucosa of the oesophagus, include radiofrequency ablation, argon plasma coagulation and less frequently photodynamic therapy. These are generally reserved for patients with dysplasia. Their place – if any – in routine clinical practice has yet to be established.

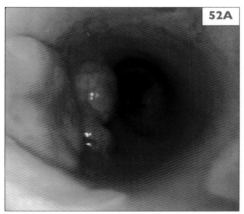
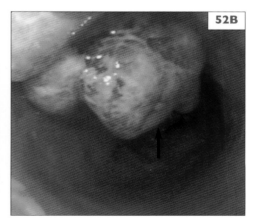

52 Two images of adenocarcinoma of the oesophagus arising in Barrett's oesophagus.

Hiatus hernia

Definition
A hiatus hernia occurs when part of the stomach leaves its normal anatomical position in the abdomen and enters the thorax. There are two forms: axial (sliding) and paraoesophageal (rolling).

Epidemiology
Axial hiatus hernias are common and are usually present in up to 50% of 50-year-olds. Paraoesophageal hernias are less common and present at a later age.

Pathophysiology
Axial (sliding) hiatus hernia
The normal relationship between oesophagus and stomach is maintained, but the cardia is displaced into the thorax (**53, 54**). Lower oesophageal sphincter function is compromised by herniation, and gastro-oesophageal reflux may occur. Transient physiological herniation when the oesophagus shortens is normal, occurring during vomiting. It has been suggested that contraction of longitudinal oesophageal smooth muscle underlies the pathogenesis of axial hiatus hernia. As stimulation of intra-abdominal structures initiates oesophageal smooth muscle contraction, this may explain the clinical associations between gallstone disease and hiatus hernia.

Paraoesophageal hiatus hernia
In paraoesophageal hiatus hernia, the gastric fundus herniates lateral to the cardia, through a diaphragmatic weakness caused by failed closure of the lateral pleuroperitoneal canal.

Clinical history
Most patients with axial hiatus hernias are asymptomatic. Classical symptoms are heartburn (pyrosis), acid regurgitation, and waterbrash. Dysphagia indicates oesophagitis or the development of stricture. Severe reflux can lead to pulmonary aspiration.

The classical symptom of paraoesophageal hernias is dysphagia that changes with posture. Heartburn is not a feature. Most patients present with vague upper gastrointestinal symptoms, or the hernia is noted as an incidental finding on chest radiography. Anaemia from intractable ulceration at the neck of the paraoesophageal hernia may occur (riding-ulcer). There is a significant risk of strangulation, obstruction of the herniated stomach, and gastric volvulus.

Physical examination
This is usually normal.

Laboratory and special examinations
Mild reflux symptoms need not be investigated. Barium radiology will demonstrate both paraoesophageal and axial hiatus hernia (**55**).

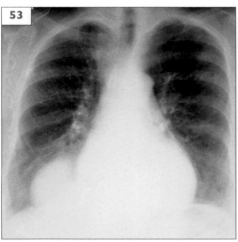

53 Plain X-ray showing hiatus hernia adjacent to right heart border.

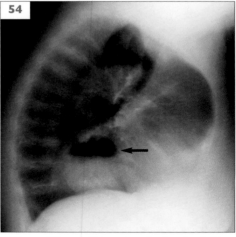

54 Lateral X-ray of hiatus hernia showing fluid level in stomach within chest.

Axial hiatus hernia can usually be seen at endoscopy, but small hernia will be reduced by intubating the stomach and so may escape notice. Negotiating a large axial hiatus hernia can be difficult at endoscopy (**56, 57**).

Management

Asymptomatic axial hiatus hernias require no treatment. If treatment is required, the general management approach is that for reflux. Those with mild reflux symptoms are advised to avoid stooping, to avoid tight-fitting garments, and to sleep with the head of the bed elevated. Frequent light meals are better tolerated than large meals. In some patients, specific foods induce symptoms and should be avoided. The value of these measures is questionable and largely untested. Patients should be advised that smoking reduces the lower oesophageal tone and is a mucosal irritant, and therefore liable to worsen symptoms. Increasingly severe symptoms should be managed with alginates, antacids, and acid suppression as for gastro-oesophageal reflux disease (GORD).

The incidence and severity of complications in paraoesophageal hiatus hernia means that all patients should be considered for surgical repair. However, because of the greater age, frailty, and comorbidity of these patients, this is often impractical. Laparoscopic and open surgical approaches are both used.

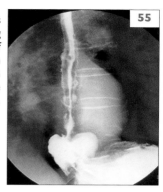

55 Hiatus hernia, showing protrusion of upper portion of stomach through the diaphragm.

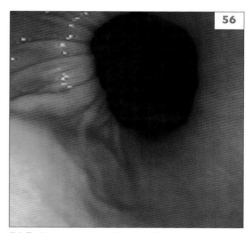

56 Endoscopic view of an axial hiatus hernia looking down from the oesophagus.

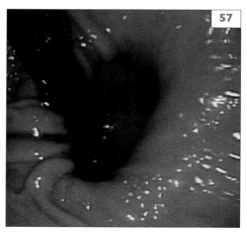

57 Mixed hiatus hernia.

Stomach and duodenum

Inflammatory diseases and neoplasia dominate gastric pathology. Neoplasia is very rare in the duodenum

***Helicobacter pylori* can cause acute and chronic gastritis, and predisposes to gastric and duodenal ulceration, gastric atrophy, and gastric cancer**

Endoscopy is the predominant diagnostic modality

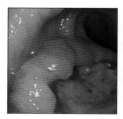
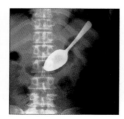
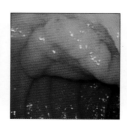
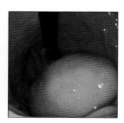

Stomach: anatomy and histology

The stomach extends from the oesophagogastric junction below the diaphragm to the pylorus (gastroduodenal junction), the latter being fixed to the peritoneum. The oesophagogastric junction may be mobile (hiatus hernia). The anatomical borders are the lesser and greater curves, but the body of the stomach is mobile and can be distorted. The stomach may be divided into the cardia, fundus, body, and antrum. The acid-producing mucosa is located predominantly in the body.

Histology

As in all other parts of the intestine, layers of gut wall consist of:

- Mucosa.
- Muscularis mucosae (thin layer of organized muscle).
- Submucosa (connective tissue).
- Circular muscle fibres.
- Longitudinal muscle fibres.
- Outer serosal lining.

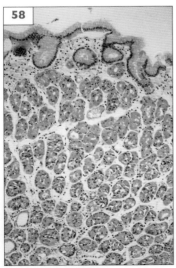

58 Normal histology of the acid-bearing area of the stomach.

The gastric mucosa is specialized for acid production, which occurs in pit-like glands lined with acid-producing cells (parietal cells) (**58**). These cells contain the proton pump. A specialized area of the glands is responsible for regenerating cells, which migrate to reform surface epithelium. The luminal surface of the gastric mucosa is covered with a mucous layer, which traps a protective layer of bicarbonate to protect mucosal cells from acid.

Gastric antral histology is different, in that there is no acid production. The antrum is responsible for the control of acid production, with a high concentration of gastrin-producing cells in the submucosa. Stimulation of gastrin following an increase in gastric pH (due to food ingestion) leads to acid release from parietal cells. When the stomach is empty and the pH falls, gastrin production is switched off. Circular and longitudinal smooth muscle activity is coordinated to allow peristaltic waves to pass the food through to the gastrointestinal tract.

Investigation of the stomach

Upper gastrointestinal symptoms are common in the general population, but lack specificity and discriminate poorly between functional disease and organic pathology. Consequently, many patients are referred for upper gastrointestinal tract investigation.

ENDOSCOPY

This is the most common investigation (**59**) and is very sensitive in detecting mucosal changes; samples from any lesion can be sent for histological or cytological assessment, and infection of the mucosa (by *H. pylori*) can be assessed. Endoscopic ultrasound (EUS) is used to characterize submucosal lesions, differentiating these from extrinsic compression, and in assessing the depth, local spread, or recurrence of gastric tumours.

There are attendant risks from sedation (especially in patients with concurrent cardiorespiratory disease), and perforation or haemorrhage following instrumentation. Although the risk is small in diagnostic endoscopy (mortality of the order of 1:10,000), it is higher in therapeutic procedures.

Postoperative stomach

Except for the immediate postoperative phase, the complications of the postsurgical stomach, such as stomal ulceration, gastritis, oesophagitis, bezoar formation, and tumour recurrence, are best assessed endoscopically.

Gastrointestinal bleeding

Emergency endoscopy in patients with upper gastrointestinal bleeding will identify the cause. In cases of peptic ulcer bleeding, endoscopic criteria will assist in stratifying the risk of rebleeding, and it is frequently possible to treat the bleeding lesion endoscopically (for example by injection therapy, or heat treatment).

RADIOLOGY

The barium meal examination is excellent for detecting anatomical variations, such as large hiatus hernias or chronic gastric volvulus, which can be bewildering to the endoscopist. Double-contrast studies can delineate mucosal lesions such as polyps, erosions, and ulcers. Although benign and malignant ulcers can be separated using radiological criteria, this is not sufficiently sensitive, and all gastric ulcers must be assessed histologically by multiple repeated biopsies at endoscopy.

Postoperative stomach

Radiological assessment is useful to investigate the early complications in the postoperative stomach. Examples include anastomotic leakage or postoperative obstruction, which are best investigated with water-soluble contrast radiology.

Gastrointestinal bleeding

The presence of lesions potentially causing upper gastrointestinal haemorrhage can be detected using contrast radiology, but whether or not they are the source of blood loss cannot be determined. Small erosions require sensitive double-contrast techniques. Barium studies have a very limited role, due to the superiority of endoscopic diagnosis and endoscopic therapy.

Motility

Barium meal examination is, however, better than endoscopy at detecting loss of antral peristalsis and antral narrowing. This occurs in diffuse infiltrative processes, such as linitis plastica from

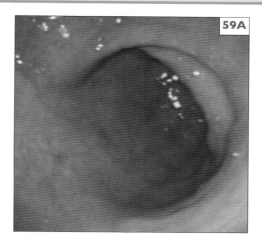

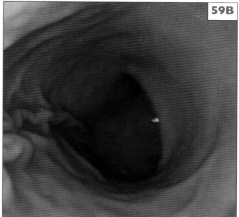

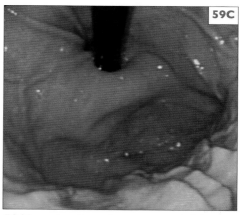

59 Normal endoscopic appearances of the stomach. (**A**) Antrum, (**B**) body, and (**C**) fundus (the endoscope is in the retroverted or 'J' position).

gastric carcinoma or lymphoma, chronic granulomatous diseases (Crohn's, tuberculosis, sarcoidosis, and syphilis), and amyloid. These can be missed at endoscopy unless a full-thickness or snare biopsy is taken.

Gastroparesis (loss of motility due to autonomic neuropathy in diabetics) and slow gastric emptying can be detected by barium meal, but are best quantitated by scintigraphy.

GASTRIC SCINTIGRAPHY

Some estimate of gastric emptying can be made by barium meal. Gastric stasis is suggested by the finding of food residue in a fasted stomach at endoscopy; however, this is best studied by gastric scintigraphy. Scintigraphic studies use a gamma-camera to follow the progress of a standard meal containing a nonabsorbable tracer (**60**). After gastric surgery, very rapid gastric emptying can occur; in some cases, food transits the stomach in 5 mins. In most patients, symptoms improve during the first 18 months postoperatively and, by using this technique, clinical progress can be monitored.

GASTRIC ACID SECRETION

In the past, gastric acid secretion was frequently studied in the investigation of patients with pernicious anaemia (who have achlorhydria) and to assess acid secretion following vagotomy for peptic ulceration. Today, it is used in research, and sometimes in the investigation of suspected Zollinger–Ellison syndrome.

Gastric contents are aspirated via a nasogastric tube in a fasted subject. Basal, unstimulated secretion is measured over 1 hr with four, 15-min samples. Gastric acid secretion is then stimulated with intravenous pentagastrin and further samples are collected. Stimulated secretion is expressed as either maximal acid output (the total 1-hr acid output after pentagastrin) or peak acid output (twice the sum of the two highest acid outputs over two consecutive 15-min collections). The maximal and peak acid outputs are a measure of parietal cell mass, which is higher in men than in women. It is increased in Zollinger–Ellison syndrome and is lower following antrectomy.

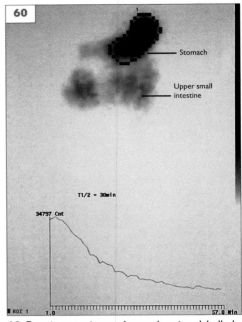

60 Gastric emptying study; a technetium-labelled meal, showing gradual emptying of the isotope from the stomach. The rate of loss can be quantified. In this example, the $t_{1/2}$ (time to half-emptying of the stomach) is 30 mins.

Zollinger–Ellison syndrome

This is a rare condition caused by a gastrin-secreting tumour (generally in the pancreas or duodenum, **61**). It can be part of the multiple endocrine neoplasia (MEN) 1 syndrome, a genetic syndrome in which gastrin-secreting tumours are associated with pituitary tumours (e.g. prolactinoma) and hyperparathyroidism. Patients present with multiple peptic ulcers extending into the distal duodenum and jejunum, as a consequence of gastrin-driven acid secretion. Diarrhoea is reported in up to one-third of patients – probably reflecting pH-dependent inhibition of pancreatic lipases.

Pathology and pathophysiology

The tumours are often multiple, most often in the pancreas. In two-thirds of patients, the tumours are malignant. Basal acid and stimulated acid secretion is raised, but there is overlap into the reference range. Hypergastrinaemia is found and, unlike normal subjects, intravenous infusion of the hormone secretin augments serum gastrin levels. As with other neuroendocrine tumours, serum chromogranin A is frequently raised.

Treatment

Acid hypersecretion is controlled medically by high-dose proton pump inhibitor treatment and, if possible, the primary tumour is excised surgically. Tumour localization can be problematic and may require EUS (for pancreatic lesions and those in the duodenal wall), angiography, and intraoperative ultrasound.

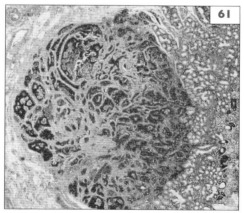

61 A gastrinoma in the wall of the duodenum, demonstrating that these tumours may be small, but may still be responsible for devastating hyperacidity.

Gastritis

Gastritis is inflammation of the gastric mucosa. Classification has been contentious, but an international working party has proposed a new scheme. The purpose was to incorporate endoscopic and biopsy findings, and to recognize the bacterium *H. pylori* as the principal cause of chronic, nonimmune gastritis. This so-called 'Sydney classification' makes a distinction between acute, chronic, and special forms of gastritis, and has a histological division and endoscopic division. The histological division covers inflammation (chronic inflammatory cells), activity (neutrophils), atrophy (diminution of gastric glands), intestinal metaplasia, and the presence of *H. pylori*. The endoscopic division describes the endoscopic appearance of the mucosa.

ACUTE GASTRITIS
Definition
This is gastric mucosal injury, leading to an acute inflammation with or without ulceration.

Pathophysiology
Acute gastritis has several causes:
- Direct gastric mucosal injury can be caused by alcohol, corrosives, drugs, and irradiation.
- Stress ulceration is associated with tissue hypoxia, hypovolaemia, major trauma, sepsis, multiorgan failure, head injury (Cushing's ulcer), and burns (Curling's ulcer). Stress ulcers arise as a result of impaired gastric mucosal blood flow, and are most frequent in the proximal part of the stomach.
- Bacterial infection such as acute food poisoning (e.g. *Staphylococcus aureus* toxins).

Clinical history and examination
Patients complain of abdominal pain, anorexia, nausea, retching, and gastrointestinal bleeding. In the setting of the intensive therapy unit (ITU) patient, these lesions are a frequent cause of GI bleeding – shallow erosions present with bleeding from the capilliary plexus.

Laboratory and special examinations
The mucosa is erythematous and congested at endoscopy. Erosions (mucosal lesions without depth), ulceration, and haemorrhage are also seen (62–64).

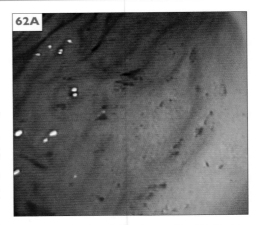

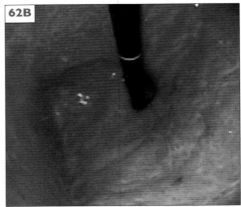

62 Haemorrhagic gastritis with mild patchy erythema: (**A**), antegrade view; (**B**) in retroversion.

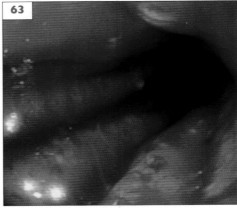

63 Severe haemorrhagic gastritis with acute gastrointestinal bleeding.

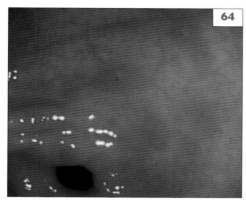

64 Small pyloric and antral erosions at endoscopy.

Special forms
Acute corrosive gastritis
This is a serious condition following ingestion of acids, alkali, or other necrotizing agents. Patients can become shocked and gastric necrosis can ensue. Management is with nasogastric aspiration, acid suppression, and surgery if necrosis develops.

Acute phlegmonous gastritis
This is a severe purulent bacterial infection of the full thickness of the gastric wall, caused by Gram-positive cocci or coliforms. The condition is rare, usually affecting patients with pre-existing mucosal disease of the stomach. The patient is systemically ill with an acute abdomen, pyrexia, leukocytosis, and purulent vomiting. Management is with antibiotics, rehydration, and surgery.

Differential diagnosis
Differentiation from other forms of gastric inflammation (e.g. chronic ulceration) and chronic gastritis is important.

Prognosis
The prognosis depends on the cause.

Management
A number of strategies can reduce stress ulceration and minimize the risk of gastrointestinal bleeding. In high-risk patients – typically in ITU – options include locally active mucosal protective agents, such as sucralfate, acid suppression regimes (H_2 receptor antagonists or proton pump inhibitors), and enteral feeding. In established disease, the mainstay of therapy is appropriate resuscitation, correction of organ failure, and treatment of sepsis.

CHRONIC GASTRITIS
Definition
Chronic gastritis encompasses the various conditions associated with chronic inflammatory infiltrate in the gastric mucosa.

Epidemiology
Endoscopy studies indicate that histological features of chronic gastritis are found in up to 50% of normal asymptomatic people.

Aetiology
The major cause of chronic gastritis is now recognized as *H. pylori* infection, which is responsible for around 80% of all cases. Idiopathic chronic gastritis accounts for 10–15%, and autoimmune chronic gastritis for about 5%. Specific, rarer forms, such as granulocytic (Crohn's, sarcoidosis, tuberculosis, and syphilis), eosinophilic, and rugal hypertrophic gastritis, account for the remainder.

Pathophysiology
H. pylori-associated chronic gastritis is discussed later in this chapter.

Clinical history
The presence of gastritis is poorly correlated with symptomatic dyspepsia. Endoscopic duodenitis and active peptic ulcer disease are more closely linked to dyspeptic symptoms.

Physical examination
There are usually no physical signs. Autoimmune chronic gastritis is often associated with other autoimmune diseases, such as vitiligo, thyroid disorders, Addison's disease, and type I diabetes mellitus, and signs of these may be evident.

Laboratory and special examinations
Endoscopy may show diffuse reddening or patchy abnormalities (**64**) but these findings are not specific. As the mucosa can be macroscopically normal in chronic gastritis, biopsy is essential for the diagnosis and to determine the cause. *H. pylori* is the most common cause of chronic gastritis, and this should be sought by histology, culture, or urease tests.

Management

Treatment is symptomatic. Antacids and acid suppression may help. *H. pylori* eradication is rarely symptomatically helpful (unless gastric or duodenal ulceration is present). Whether *H. pylori* should be eradicated in an attempt to prevent subsequent development of gastric cancer is controversial and unproven.

AUTOIMMUNE CHRONIC GASTRITIS

Epidemiology

Autoimmune chronic gastritis is more common in women than in men (3:1), and is associated with northern European ancestry and the genetic haplotype HLA-B8 and DR3.

Pathophysiology

Autoimmune chronic gastritis causes an antral-sparing atrophic gastritis with hypergastrinaemia. Parietal cell destruction is assumed to be a consequence of lymphocytic infiltration; the proton pump is one of the antigens recognized by parietal cell autoantibodies. As the corpus mucosa becomes atrophic and thinned in advanced disease, gastric acidity falls. As a result, gastrin-producing neuroendocrine G-cells respond by producing high levels of gastrin, leading to hypergastrinaemia.

Laboratory and special examinations

Serological findings

Parietal cell autoantibodies are present in the serum of 90% of patients with autoimmune chronic gastritis; intrinsic factor antibodies occur in the minority (<20%) of patients, who are likely to progress to pernicious anaemia. In established pernicious anaemia, serum vitamin B_{12} levels are low. Following ingestion of labelled vitamin B_{12}, <10% is excreted in the urine within 24 hr, but this is corrected when ingestion of B_{12} is repeated with intrinsic factor (this is the basis of the Schilling test).

Histology

Unlike *H. pylori*-associated gastritis, autoimmune chronic gastritis is inactive (no polymorphonuclear leukocytes). There is an increased risk of epithelial dysplasia and gastric cancer (approximately three-fold). Hyperplastic and adenomatous gastric polyps are also more common. Rarely, multiple benign gastric carcinoid tumours may arise as a consequence of hypergastrinaemia, which stimulates proliferation of the enterochromaffin-like cells in the mucosa.

Differential diagnosis

Autoimmune chronic gastritis should be differentiated from acute gastritis and chronic ulceration.

Prognosis

The condition may predispose to gastric cancer, but is often asymptomatic and nonprogressive.

Management

Pernicious anaemia is treated with injections of vitamin B_{12} (1,000 µg every 2–3 months). Endoscopic surveillance for the early detection of gastric cancer in pernicious anaemia is controversial.

Helicobacter pylori

H. pylori is now recognized as the major acquired factor in the aetiology of duodenal ulcer disease, revising the aetiology, pathophysiology, and management of peptic ulcer disease.

H. pylori is a curved or spiral flagellated, Gram-negative microaerophilic bacterium. Despite the original classification as *Campylobacter*-like, it has no relationship to these organisms, and is not linked to *Campylobacter* infections elsewhere in the gastrointestinal tract. The specific feature of *H. pylori* that allows it to adapt to the acid medium of the stomach is its ability to generate local alkali (ammonia) by splitting urea with its specific urease enzyme.

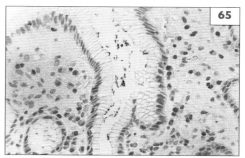

65 *H. pylori* seen at the surface of the gastric epithelium.

Epidemiology

H. pylori infection occurs worldwide and is usually acquired in childhood. Infection is more prevalent in lower socioeconomic groups, as risk factors include poor living standards (such as crowded living conditions). In developed countries, the prevalence is low in children, but rises with increasing age, paralleling the age-related prevalence of chronic gastritis (20% of 20-year-olds and 60% of 60-year-olds). In poorer communities, the prevalence is high in all age groups.

TYPES OF *H. PYLORI* INFECTION

Acute *H. pylori* infection

Little is known about the acute phase of *H. pylori* infection. A short-lived illness with epigastric pain, nausea, and vomiting associated with hypochlorhydria has been reported following ingestion of *H. pylori*. It is not known how frequently acute symptoms occur during the acquisition of *H. pylori*, or what determines the outcome of acute infection. The consequences of chronic *H. pylori* infection are more important in clinical practice.

Chronic *H. pylori* infection

H. pylori colonizes the epithelium of the gastric antrum in chronic infection (**65**). The organism lies adjacent to the gastric epithelial cells, and in the gastric pits beneath the mucous layer. Active, chronic gastritis develops predominantly in the antrum. Degenerative changes occur in the epithelium, and chronic inflammatory cells consisting of polymorphs, plasma cells, and lymphocytes infiltrate the mucosa. Lymphoid aggregation and follicle formation also occur in the basal mucosa. Following eradication of the *H. pylori* infection, these features regress – the polymorph infiltrate resolves rapidly and the lymphocytic infiltrate more slowly. In continuing infection, the histological changes are not static; over decades, they can progress from gastritis to atrophy. In some patients, this eventually leads to intestinal metaplasia. It is uncertain if eradication during these later stages of infection influences the histological changes.

The most severe gastritis is seen in young to middle-aged adults, whereas atrophic changes develop later in the disease process in older people. As gastric glands atrophy, the number of *H. pylori* organisms falls as, paradoxically, this mucosa supports the organism less well. Finally, intestinal metaplasia develops with the appearance of villiform structures and intestinal architecture. Advanced intestinal metaplasia is a factor in the development of gastric cancer.

Diagnosis

Invasive/endoscopic methods

The importance of *H. pylori* infection to upper gastrointestinal disease means that it is convenient to diagnose it at endoscopy. However, there are no specific endoscopic features of *H. pylori* infection.

Histological assessment

Histological assessment of an endoscopic antral biopsy is a reliable means of detecting *H. pylori*, but is expensive, requires expertise, and the result is not immediately available.

Culture

Culture of endoscopic biopsies is equally sensitive and specific, but suffers similar drawbacks.

Urease tests

Several methods rely on the enzyme urease for *H. pylori* detection. Incubation of an infected antral biopsy in a solution of urea generates ammonia by enzymatic degradation. The alkaline pH is visualized by a colour change in an indicator. Although sensitivity is less than biopsy or culture, urease tests have the advantage of convenience, simplicity, and speed (a rapid version of the test can be read in 1 min). False negative results can occur in patients with gastrointestinal bleeding, proton pump inhibitor therapy, or recent antibiotic treatment (**66**).

Noninvasive tests

Breath tests

The liberation of carbon dioxide in breath following urea ingestion can be used as a marker of *H. pylori* infection. Fasting subjects ingest isotopically labelled urea. In the *H. pylori*-

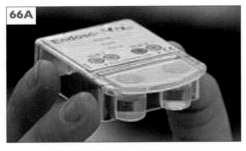

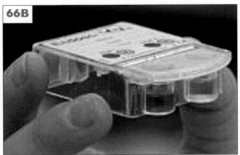

66 Urease test: (**A**) negative; (**B**) positive. This is one of a number of commercially available systems. Gastric biopsies are incubated in the chamber and the urease induces a pH change detected as a change in the indicator.

colonized stomach, the organism catabolizes the urea to release carbon dioxide, which is absorbed and excreted in the breath. After an interval, breath is collected and the labelled carbon dioxide measured. Either ^{13}C- or ^{14}C-labelled urea is used. ^{13}C is a stable nonradioactive isotope, and measurement requires a mass spectrometer. ^{14}C is radioactive, and is detectable by scintillation counter. Since these tests also rely on urease, they too can give false negative results with patients taking proton pump inhibitor therapy or after a recent course of antibiotics.

Urea breath tests are also used in assessing *H. pylori* status after an attempt at *H. pylori* eradication.

H. pylori serology

Antibodies to *H. pylori* antigens can be detected by enzyme-linked immunosorbent assay (ELISA), and are indicative of current or past infection. Although in an individual patient, antibody titres do fall slowly after successful *H. pylori* eradication, this is not helpful in assessing the success of eradication therapy.

Faecal *H. pylori* antigen detection has been described both for diagnosis of *H. pylori* colonization and for assessment of eradication.

Disease associations with *H. pylori*

Duodenal ulcer

There is a very strong association between chronic *H. pylori* infection and the development of duodenal ulceration. Up to 95% of patients with duodenal ulceration have evidence of *H. pylori* infection. However, it is important to recall that *H. pylori* infection is very common in the general population.

Gastric ulceration

H. pylori infection is also strongly linked to the development of gastric ulcers, although not as closely as duodenal ulcers. Around 75–80% of gastric ulcer patients are infected.

Gastric cancer

The aetiology of gastric cancer is multifactorial and incompletely understood. Before the current interest in *H. pylori*, it was appreciated that gastric cancers often arose in areas of intestinal metaplasia and gastric atrophy. It has been suggested that *H. pylori* infection might facilitate the progression of changes from gastritis to gastric atrophy to intestinal metaplasia to gastric cancer. This hypothesis is based on the association between *H. pylori* infection rates shown by seroepidemiology and gastric cancer rates in different populations, and evidence of past *H. pylori* infection in patients with gastric cancer.

Mucosa-associated lymphoid tissue lymphomas (MALTomas)

MALTomas – B-cell lymphomas of the gastric mucosa – have been described in *H. pylori* infection. These are rare and, for low-grade lesions, there are reports of tumour regression with *H. pylori* eradication.

H. pylori and dyspepsia

Dyspeptic symptoms are prevalent in the general population, as is *H. pylori* colonization, but the relationship between these events is complex. There is strong evidence that *H. pylori* colonization confers risk of peptic ulcer disease, and this is attenuated with eradication therapy. However, studies of *H. pylori* eradication in dyspeptic patients have generally been disappointing. Using symptomatic relief as an end point, *H. pylori* eradication in patients with uninvestigated uncomplicated dyspepsia confers a small benefit. There is an even smaller effect on dyspeptic symptoms of *H. pylori* eradication in those patients in whom endoscopy fails to demonstrate peptic ulcer disease (so-called 'endoscopy-negative' dyspepsia or nonulcer dyspepsia). Strategies promoting noninvasive tests to diagnose *H. pylori* colonization in patients with uncomplicated dyspepsia and subsequent *H. pylori* eradication therapy have been termed 'test and treat'. This has been advocated as a cost-effective approach to the management of uncomplicated dyspepsia in young patients.

Other associations

There are other associations with *H. pylori* infection, including the finding that *H. pylori*-infected children are smaller than their uninfected peers.

TREATMENT

The ideal treatment for *H. pylori* would be simple, highly effective, lacking in side effects, and cheap. This has proved difficult to achieve in practice, partly because of the ecological niche that *H. pylori* occupies, partly because of resistance to antibiotics, and partly because the acid pH of the stomach is far from optimal for antibiotic activity.

Eradication regimes are under constant review. Currently, antibiotic combinations (or combinations of antibiotics with acid suppression), over different time scales, give high rates of eradication – defined as absent *H. pylori* 4 weeks after treatment has finished. With 'triple therapy' (high-dose proton pump inhibition with two antibiotics), eradication rates reach 80–90%, providing that the patient is compliant with the multi-tablet regime. Dual therapy (using a proton pump inhibitor with a single antibiotic) is associated with poorer eradication rates compared to triple therapy. In Europe, there are concerns regarding resistance to metronidazole and, to a lesser degree, other antibiotics. Second-line therapies (for treatment failures) with quadruple therapy include combinations of proton pump inhibitors, bismuth, tetracycline, and metronidazole.

The indications for treating *H. pylori* infection are also in flux. *H. pylori*-associated peptic ulceration is universally accepted as an indication to eradicate *H. pylori*, and successful eradication will prevent disease recurrence. *H. pylori* eradication has been advocated in patients with MALToma, a positive family history of gastric cancer, and, by some, if patients will require long-term proton pump inhibitor therapy.

Chronic gastric ulcers

Definition
Chronic ulcers of the stomach are areas of mucosal ulceration extending to a variable (>1 mm) degree into the submucosal tissues. They can be complicated by perforation and haemorrhage.

Epidemiology
The lifetime prevalence of gastric ulcer is 3% in females and 4% in males. Among the elderly, it may be more common in women. The median age at presentation is 50–60 years, about a decade after the peak incidence of duodenal ulceration.

Pathophysiology
The pathogenesis of gastric ulceration is poorly understood. *H. pylori* is associated with 75–85% of gastric ulcers, a lower proportion than in duodenal ulceration. Also, basal and peak acid output is lower in patients with gastric ulcers than in those with duodenal ulcers, probably because of the associated atrophic gastritis. Smoking is a risk factor.

Clinical history
Gastric ulcers can occur without symptoms. Symptomatic patients complain of attacks of epigastric pain lasting hours and often coming in cycles that last 6–8 weeks; the attacks may then abate for several months. Symptoms can be exacerbated by food. These complaints are nonspecific and a variety of other upper gastrointestinal symptoms are reported, so that gastric ulcer cannot be differentiated from other causes of dyspepsia on clinical grounds.

Physical examination
Epigastric tenderness is found in some patients.

Laboratory and special examinations
Endoscopy and biopsy is the primary diagnostic modality (**67**). Barium studies continue to have a role (**68**), but any ulcer diagnosed in this way must still be biopsied. Gastric ulcers are found most frequently on the lesser curve at the junction between the antrum and body mucosa, as an oval or round lesion with slough-covered base. All gastric ulcers must be biopsied in each quadrant and floor, to differentiate them from malignant ulcers. Concurrent endoscopic brushing for cytological assessment increases diagnostic

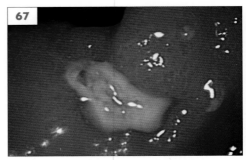

67 Benign gastric ulcer located at the incisura of the stomach.

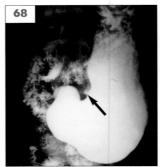

68 Barium meal showing benign gastric ulcer at incisura (arrowed).

accuracy. *H. pylori* should be sought, as this is more prevalent in gastric ulcer patients compared with controls.

A repeat endoscopic assessment is usually scheduled about 8 weeks after the index procedure, to confirm that the ulcer has healed.

Special forms
NSAID ulcers
NSAIDs inhibit gastric prostaglandin synthesis, and impair gastroduodenal mucosal defences and ulcer healing. Acute ingestion is associated with acute gastric erosions, followed by an adaptive response over 1–2 months. Ulcers associated with chronic ingestion of NSAIDs are often asymptomatic, until complicated by perforation or bleeding.

Resistant ulcers
Ulcers failing to heal after 8 weeks of treatment with acid suppression therapy are termed resistant. Biopsies should be repeated to be certain that the ulcer is not malignant. Surgery is

indicated if the ulcer fails to heal after a further course of therapy.

Differential diagnosis

Between 4 and 10% of gastric ulcers are malignant, and so gastric cancer must be excluded in all gastric ulcers. Rolled irregular ulcer margins suggest malignancy (**69**), and ulcers >2 cm are four times more likely to be malignant than smaller ulcers. Endoscopy and biopsy must be repeated until the ulcer is healed.

Prognosis

Up to two-thirds of gastric ulcers will recur in 1 year.

MANAGEMENT

General management

Smoking reduces ulcer healing and so should be discouraged. Diet makes no difference to healing rates.

Drug therapy

Acid suppression

Acid suppression has proved very successful in treating gastric ulcers. Healing rates are related to length of treatment and to the degree of 24-hr acid suppression, but after 8 weeks of treatment, 80–90% of ulcers will be healed. Proton pump inhibitors are more potent at suppressing gastric acid than H_2 receptor antagonists, which can also be used. Side effects limit the usefulness of anticholinergic drugs.

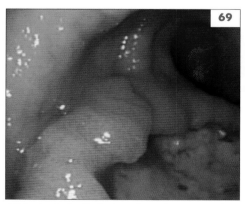

69 A classical rolled edge of a malignant gastric ulcer – this was an antral cancer.

Mucosal protective agents

Prostaglandins are important in regulating mucosal blood flow, re-epithelialization after injury, and mucus secretion. Misoprostol is a synthetic prostaglandin E_2 analogue that has mucosal protective and antisecretory activity, and is active in treating gastric ulcers. It is also used in attenuating the gastroduodenal damage of NSAIDs; the side effects include diarrhoea. Sucralfate, an aluminium salt of sucrose octasulphate, is a surface-acting agent that binds to the base of ulcers. It may stimulate mucosal prostaglandins, and can be used to treat gastric ulcers. In clinical practice, these agents have been eclipsed by the more effective proton pump inhibitors.

H. pylori eradication

H. pylori should be eradicated, although the importance of this in patients with gastric ulcer is less clear than in duodenal ulcer disease.

Maintenance acid suppression therapy

As gastric ulceration is frequently recurrent and may be asymptomatic, maintenance acid suppression therapy is often considered. This is indicated for large (>2 cm) ulcers, patients with a history of previous ulcers, those who need to continue NSAIDs, and elderly patients or those with concurrent cardiorespiratory disease, which would make them particularly vulnerable in the event of an ulcer-related complication.

Surgery

Surgery was once common for peptic ulceration, but now is rare in the elective setting. Indications for surgery are:

- Presence of complications (perforation, bleeding).
- Resistant ulcers.
- Suspicion of malignancy.
- Ulcers that relapse on maintenance therapy.

The usual operation is a Bilroth I partial gastrectomy, which reduces the parietal cell mass, but leaves the normal pathway of food from stomach to duodenum unchanged. Occasionally, a Polya gastrectomy is performed (see 'Complications of gastric surgery', for a fuller description of these procedures).

Gastric cancer

Definition
Gastric cancer is primary cancer of the stomach.

Epidemiology
Gastric carcinoma is a common cancer of the upper gastrointestinal tract. The incidence peaks between the ages of 55 and 65 years, and men are affected twice as often as women.

There are geographic variations in the disease prevalence, the cause of which is unknown. Chile and Japan, for instance, have especially high rates. Incidence of gastric cancer in the distal stomach is declining, in contrast to cancers of the proximal stomach, gastro-oesophageal junction, and oesophagus.

Aetiology
The aetiology of gastric cancer is multifactorial and a variety of factors have been implicated.

Dietary habits
N-nitrosamine compounds are derived from dietary nitrates and nitrites by bacterial action, and are directly carcinogenic. Diets rich in vitamins A, E, and C are protective.

Environmental carcinogens
These include alcohol and cigarette smoking.

Genetic factors
Carriage of blood group A confers increased risk and there is a (minor) familial tendency. Risk is increased in patients with familial adenomatous polyposis and some forms of hereditary non-polyposis colorectal cancer.

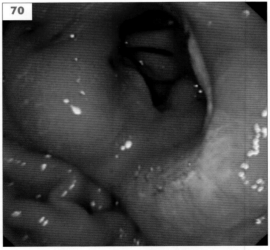

70 Gastric cancer arising many years after partial gastrectomy for peptic ulcer disease.

H. pylori infection

There is increasing evidence that acquisition of *H. pylori* at an early age is a risk factor in the development of gastric carcinoma. Chronic atrophic gastritis with intestinal metaplasia is recognized as a predisposing factor for gastric cancer, and is also associated with *H. pylori* infection. Intestinal metaplasia type III (colonic type), associated with sulfo-mucin producing goblet cells, is more strongly implicated than either of the other types.

Adenomatous polyps

These are uncommon, but have malignant potential.

Previous gastric surgery

An increased incidence of gastric cancer is apparent 15–20 years after partial gastrectomy (**70**).

Other factors

Patients with pernicious anaemia and achlorhydria have a small but increased risk of gastric cancer.

Pathophysiology

Macroscopic appearances range from ulceration (**69**), to polypoid lesions, to diffuse infiltrative lesions (linitis plastica, **71**, **72**). Ulcerative forms are most common, generally in the antrum and lesser curve. About 95% are adenocarcinomas and arise in areas of intestinal metaplasia.

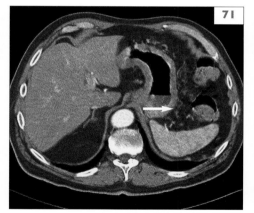

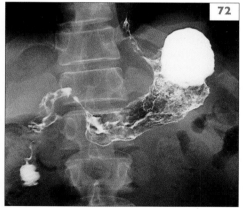

71 CT scan of linitis plastica – the gastric wall is very thickened and undistended.

72 Barium meal showing gastric cancer of the linitis plastica type – this constricted stomach wall is diffusely infiltrated and the stomach cannot dilate.

The cancer may spread directly into adjacent structures or via the regional lymphatics, which eventually drain into the cisterna chyli and thoracic duct. Peritoneal spread is common, and ovarian deposits (Krukenberg tumours) may occur (73–75).

Clinical history

Symptoms are often vague in the early stages. There are no features to distinguish dyspepsia associated with gastric cancer from benign causes, but the history is usually short (<1 year). Anorexia and weight loss are common as the disease advances. Haematemesis occurs, but is unusual. Early satiety may be a prominent feature of diffuse infiltrating carcinoma (linitis plastica), due to immobility of the stomach wall. Gastric outlet obstruction may be a late feature of advanced antral carcinoma, with nausea and vomiting.

Physical examination

In patients with disease confined to the stomach, there are no physical signs. However, 25% of patients present with metastatic disease in the lungs, liver, bone, and brain. Evidence of metastases may be detected clinically – including Troisier's sign, indicating involvement of the supraclavicular nodes. Nonmetastatic manifestations include acanthosis nigricans, thrombophlebitis migrans (Trousseau's sign), and dermatomyositis.

Laboratory and special investigations

Diagnosis

Gastric cancer is usually suspected at gastroscopy. Endoscopic biopsies are always indicated following radiological diagnosis of gastric ulcer, to confirm or refute malignancy. Multiple biopsies and brushing are required from each quadrant of the ulcer to ensure that the diagnosis is not missed.

Staging

CT scanning, ultrasound, and bone scan are used to detect metastatic disease. CT is better at detecting hepatic metastatic disease, while EUS is occasionally valuable in assessing local lymph node involvement (nodes in the mediastinum, gastrohepatic space and coeliac axis) and tumour depth. Direct laparoscopic visualization of the peritoneum and cytology of lavage fluid may be important in selecting patients for surgery.

Special forms

'Early' gastric cancer is a term used to denote gastric cancer that is curable and recognizable endoscopically, although endoscopic changes may be very subtle. Lesions are confined to the mucosa but, paradoxically, may have venous metastases. In Japan, 5-year survival rates of 90% have been reported using limited barium meal or endoscopy in mass screening programmes to detect 'early' gastric cancer. Some of these lesions have been successfully treated by endoscopic mucosal resection.

Differential diagnosis

As the symptoms of gastric cancer in the early, curable, stage are nonspecific, it is imperative that the diagnosis is considered in all dyspeptic patients presenting in their middle years or older. Equally, since benign and malignant gastric ulcers can have identical macroscopic appearances, all gastric ulcers must be biopsied repeatedly in different sites, and followed up endoscopically until healed, in order to avoid misdiagnosis.

Prognosis

Overall, the 5-year survival rate is 10%. For inoperable disease, the mean interval from diagnosis to death is 4 months. Histological tumour grade and spread are prognostic.

Management

Surgery

This offers the only potentially curative treatment in selected patients. Curative surgery includes excision of the tumour, omentum, and lymphatics draining the area. Surgical palliation should be considered for obstruction, haemorrhage, and pain.

Chemotherapy

Patients treated surgically with curative intent are offered perioperative chemotherapy, or postoperative chemoradiotherapy.

Other treatments

Dyspeptic symptoms may respond to acid suppression, but eventually opiates are usually required for pain. Individual symptoms can be palliated in varying ways – radiotherapy (pain, bleeding, and obstruction), therapeutic endoscopic interventions (bleeding, laser and argon-plasma coagulation, or endoluminal stent to alleviate gastric outlet obstruction or dysphagia). Palliative chemotherapy has a place for some patients.

Liaison with family, the family practitioner, and palliative care specialists is important in the terminal stages.

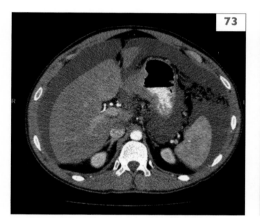

73 CT showing ascites from gastric cancer.

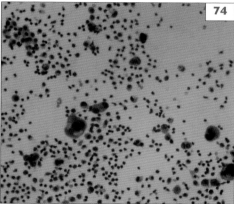

74 Clumps of adenocarcinoma cells in the ascites from **73**.

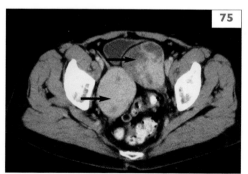

75 CT scan – the bilateral enlarged ovaries are secondary deposits from a gastric cancer (Krukenberg syndrome).

Complications of gastric surgery

Gastric surgery (76) was once commonplace. However, with the decline in peptic ulcer disease and newer pharmacological approaches to its management, and the recognition of the value of *H. pylori* eradication in preventing ulcer recurrence, this has changed.

Similar complications are shared by all types of gastric surgery, but their respective frequency varies with different operations. Most patients have some symptoms but, in general, these improve during the first 6–12 months after surgery.

STOMACH, MARGINAL OR ANASTOMOTIC ULCERS

Ulceration may occur at anastomotic sites where acid-producing gastric mucosa is directly adjacent to duodenal or small-intestinal mucosa (77). Symptoms are similar to those of any peptic ulcer. Acid reduction by H_2 antagonists or proton pump inhibitors will help, but reoperation may be necessary to further reduce acid production.

EARLY DUMPING

Rapid emptying of gastric contents into the small bowel causes symptoms of abdominal pain, diarrhoea, nausea, and systemic symptoms of faintness, sweating, and palpitations within 30 mins of eating. Three mechanisms are proposed:

- Intestinal distension may initiate autonomic reflexes that cause symptoms.
- Hyperosmolar stomach contents lead to a swift osmotic transfer of fluid out of the vascular compartment into the gut lumen, and transient hypovolaemia.
- Release of gastrointestinal hormones.

Early dumping is managed by advising small, low-carbohydrate meals taken frequently with liquid. Guar may reduce symptoms. Further surgical intervention is reserved for intractable symptoms persisting for more than a year after operation.

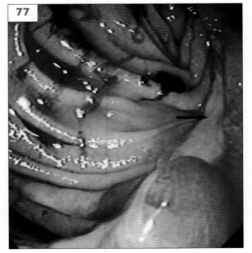

76 Diagram of main gastric operations. (**A**) Bilroth I partial gastrectomy. (**B**) Polya or Bilroth II partial gastrectomy. (**C**) Gastrojejunostomy. (**D**) Pyloroplasty. For benign disease, operations would either reduce the amount of acid-secreting mucosa (**A, B**), or drain the stomach after vagotomy (**C, D**) (since cutting the vagus to reduce acid results in a nonfunctioning pylorus).

(Labels within diagram 76:) Removal of much of body, antrum and pylorus; Jejunum; Efferent loop; Afferent loop (second part of duodenum onwards)

77 A stomal ulcer seen at endoscopy. The patient has had a Polya gastrectomy with afferent and efferent loops, and the ulcer is at the margin of the gastric and small-intestinal mucosa.

Paradoxically, gastric stasis can also be a sequel to gastric surgery. This is usually because of impaired drainage following vagotomy. The procedure of truncal vagotomy to reduce acid is always accompanied by a gastric drainage procedure (pyloroplasty or gastroenterostomy) to aid drainage.

LATE DUMPING
Rapid absorption of carbohydrate may cause an inappropriate release of insulin from the pancreas, and faintness and dizziness due to reactive hypoglycaemia 1–2 hr after eating. Treatment is similar to that for early dumping.

DIARRHOEA
This may occur due to changes in motility and rapid fluid transfer through the small intestine and colon. Symptoms occur within 1–2 hr of eating. Treatment is as for early dumping. Some patients benefit from antidiarrhoeal agents or bile salt binding with cholestyramine.

BILIOUS VOMITING
Loss of the antropyloric barrier may allow reflux of duodenal contents into the stomach. Bile and pancreatic enzymes are irritant and cause gastritis.

The endoscopic appearance has been termed the 'red and green' stomach – friable erythematous mucosa with green bilious fluid. Patients complain of pain, and may vomit bile-stained fluid. The management includes bile acid-binding agents (e.g. cholestyramine) and prokinetic agents. Reflux gastropathy is independent of the postsurgical gastritis and stomal ulceration (**77**) seen commonly at endoscopy in postsurgical stomachs.

GASTRO-OESOPHAGEAL REFLUX
Lower oesophageal sphincter tone is reduced after gastric surgery, both directly due to vagotomy, as well as due to loss of normal reflex and hormonal responses to eating. Bile reflux may also contribute.

CANCER IN THE REMNANT STOMACH
The absolute risk and mechanism is debated, but following gastric surgery the risk of gastric cancer is increased (**70**).

METABOLIC COMPLICATIONS AFTER GASTRIC SURGERY
Anaemia
Iron deficiency is common due to stomal ulceration, postsurgical gastritis, and reduced iron absorption. Megaloblastic anaemia due to vitamin B_{12} deficiency, as a result of reduction in intrinsic factor and therefore ileal malabsorption of vitamin B_{12}, may occur after a delay of many years.

Osteomalacia
This is also more common from calcium and vitamin D deficiency.

Weight loss
Weight loss after surgery is almost inevitable. It occurs because of inadequate food intake (partly because of dietary changes necessitated by dumping and diarrhoea) and malabsorption. The cause of malabsorption is not well understood, but mild degrees of steatorrhoea are common. Both bacterial overgrowth and disordered motility may contribute.

Disorders of gastric motility and bezoars

Definition
The normal stomach has rhythmic contractions, which both control and propel the boluses of food entering the small intestine. This is disturbed in a number of disease states.

Epidemiology and aetiology
See 'Special forms and complications'.

Pathophysiology
As food enters the stomach, the gastric fundus relaxes to accommodate it, after which peristaltic waves push it down to the antrum. The peristaltic process is mediated by vagal reflexes and the local intrinsic gastric plexuses.

Vagotomy or partial gastrectomy impairs accommodation, resulting in inability to consume large meals, and leads to rapid gastric emptying.

Impaired emptying results from deregulated or disordered peristalsis, and leads to delayed gastric emptying. Disordered peristalsis may underlie the development of gastric diverticulae.

Clinical history
Impaired accommodation
Patients complain of early satiety and postprandial fullness.

Rapid early emptying

This gives rise to dumping and postprandial diarrhoea, and is seen as a complication of gastric surgery.

Delayed gastric emptying

Patients experience upper abdominal pain, fullness, nausea, and vomiting. The vomiting can be projectile, and food ingested many hours or even several days previously may be seen in the vomitus. Delayed gastric emptying may occur due to conditions distorting anatomy (e.g. pyloric stenosis, antral cancer) or because of a disorder affecting neural function (e.g. diabetes). In some cases, the cause is unknown.

Physical examination

In those with delayed gastric emptying, there may be evidence of weight loss, the dilated stomach can be palpable, and there is sometimes a succussion splash (audible splash over stomach on shaking the abdomen).

Laboratory and special examinations

Barium radiology will detect food debris in the stomach and give an estimate of emptying, but scintigraphic measures of gastric emptying following a standard meal with a radiolabelled tracer offer the most sensitive test. Endoscopy is usually required to exclude mechanical

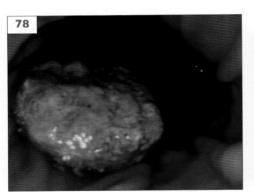

78 Phytobezoar seen at endoscopy. Phytobezoars can be broken up at endoscopy and removed.

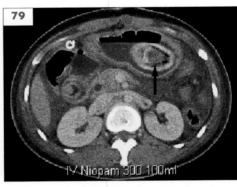

79 Bezoars seen on CT in the stomach and duodenum.

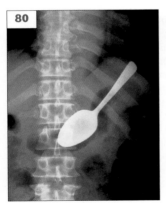

80 Ingested spoon in the stomach seen by X-ray.

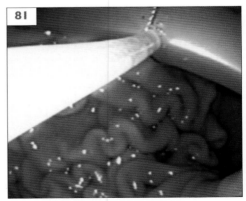

81 Ingested foreign body – pictures of a toothbrush being retrieved from the stomach at endoscopy.

obstruction, ideally after nasogastric drainage of gastric contents. Aspiration of >150 ml fluid from the stomach after an overnight fast is suggestive of delayed gastric emptying.

Special forms and complications
Bezoars
Stasis predisposes to gastric bezoars (**78, 79**) – aggregates of indigestible material, which form residue trapped in the antrum. Phytobezoars are made of concretions of fibrous vegetable material, but bezoars made of a number of other materials have been described. Trichobezoars are made of hair and food debris, and are most common in young women who habitually eat hair. Some patients who ingest hair are psychiatrically disturbed, and can also ingest various other foreign bodies (**80, 81**).

Patients present with pain, nausea, and fullness. The bezoar may be palpable, and can be confirmed by barium meal or endoscopy. Complications include gastritis, ulceration, and anaemia due to insidious bleeding.

Management consists of endoscopic disintegration of the bezoar and treating the impaired motility.

Gastroparesis and diabetic gastroparesis
Gastroparesis is diagnosed in patients with delayed gastric emptying, in whom a physical obstructing cause has been excluded. It is frequently a manifestation of diabetic autonomic neuropathy involving the vagal nerve and intrinsic plexuses of the stomach. The typical symptoms are delayed gastric emptying and, because food is delivered erratically to the duodenum, poor diabetic control. Often symptoms vary from week to week. Treatment consists of optimizing diabetic control, and the use of prokinetic agents. Erythromycin (a motilin agonist) has also been advocated. Developments such as local botulinum toxin injection to relax the pylorus in patients with pyloric spasm, and the use of electrical stimulation (gastric pacemakers), are still under consideration.

Gastric volvulus
In individuals with long, thin stomachs, rotation around the long axis of the stomach may occur (**82**). This presents with severe pain, and vomiting with only low volumes of vomitus. It often settles spontaneously, but surgical intervention may be needed.

Differential diagnosis
Mechanical obstruction of the gastric outlet causes delayed gastric emptying. In adults, this is most commonly due to pyloric stenosis by peptic ulcer disease or carcinoma. Adult hypertrophic pyloric stenosis is rare.

Delayed gastric emptying can be due to drugs such as opiates, and drugs with anticholinergic effects, such as tricyclic antidepressants. It is also common in patients with gastro-oesophageal reflux. Up to 50% of patients with nonulcer dyspepsia have delayed gastric emptying, but the relationship of this to symptoms is unclear.

Dermatomyositis, scleroderma, and myotonic muscular dystrophy are also causes of abnormal gastric motility.

Prognosis
The prognosis depends on the cause. It is poor in diabetic gastroparesis, since it usually occurs in association with autonomic neuropathy and other complications of long-standing diabetes.

Management
Prokinetic drugs such as metoclopramide or domperidone should be tried.

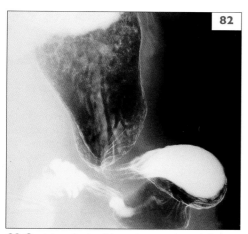

82

82 Gastric volvulus. Note the rotation of the stomach around its long axis.

Ménétrier's disease and other rugal hyperplastic gastropathies

Definition
The rugal hyperplastic gastropathies comprise a group of poorly understood diseases, in which giant gastric folds (rugae) are found at endoscopy or on radiological evaluation.

Epidemiology and aetiology
Ménétrier's disease
This is a rare condition, which may occur at any age and affects men more than women. The aetiology is unknown, although expression of the growth factor TGF-alpha is prominent in the gastric tissue.

Zollinger–Ellison syndrome
This is a rare sporadic or genetic condition in which rugal hypertrophy occurs as a response to excess production of the hormone gastrin by a neuroendocrine tumour, often located in the pancreas or duodenum.

Hypertrophic hypersecretory gastritis
This too is a rare condition with giant folds and high acid secretion, but is not associated with neuroendocrine tumours.

Pathophysiology
The characteristic macroscopic feature of Ménétrier's disease is mucus-covered giant cerebriform rugae, especially in the fundus (**83**). There may be haemorrhage and erosions associated with areas of rugal hypertrophy. The key histological features are mucous cell hyperplasia, and cystic dilatation of gastric glands submucosally. Gastric acidity is reduced as a consequence of gland atrophy and excess mucus, and protein loss occurs from the stomach.

Clinical history
The patient may give a history of indigestion.

Physical examination
There is peripheral oedema and, in severe protein loss, ascites may be present.

Laboratory and special investigations
The diagnosis is suggested by finding enlarged tortuous rugae in the corpus and greater curve of the stomach. Large endoscopic biopsies are required to examine the gland architecture. Blood investigations may reveal hypoproteinaemia. Protein loss can be documented by retrieval of labelled albumin from gastric aspirates, but is rarely performed.

Differential diagnosis
Ménétrier's disease is differentiated from gastric carcinoma and lymphoma by endoscopic biopsy and EUS. Giant rugae are also a feature of hypertrophic hypersecretory gastropathy, but this is associated with increased gastric acid secretion and normogastrinaemia. In Zollinger–Ellison syndrome, there is rugal hypertrophy, hypergastrinaemia causing parietal cell hyperplasia, and consequent excess acid leading to peptic ulceration and diarrhoea.

Prognosis
Ménétrier's disease usually runs a protracted course.

Management
There is no specific therapy for Ménétrier's disease. Acid suppression with H_2 receptor antagonists, proton pump inhibitors, or anticholinergic drugs has been tried. Surgery is reserved for patients with persistent hypoproteinaemia, blood loss, and refractory symptoms. For hypertrophic hypersecretory gastritis and Zollinger–Ellison syndrome, acid suppression is the mainstay of the treatment.

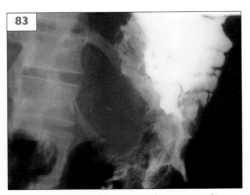

83 Giant gastric folds seen on barium meal in Ménétrier's disease (a source of protein loss).

Gastric antral vascular ectasia (synonym 'watermelon stomach')

Definition
Gastric antral vascular ectasia is diffuse vascular ectasia of the stomach antrum.

Epidemiology and aetiology
The condition is more common in females (typically, a female:male ratio of 8:1), frequently middle aged and with an autoimmune or connective tissue condition. In up to one-third of patients, there is an association with cirrhosis, and it can be a manifestation of portal hypertensive gastropathy and reduced serum gastrin levels.

Pathophysiology
The lesions are dilated ectatic vessels surrounded by fibrosis. In cirrhosis, they may develop from intramural vascular shunts caused by portal hypertension.

Clinical history
Patients present with overt or covert gastrointestinal bleeding.

Physical examination
There may be evidence of anaemia and signs of cirrhosis.

Laboratory and special investigations
The diagnosis is usually made at endoscopy. Typically, red/blue lesions are clustered on the crests of longitudinal rugal folds that converge on the pylorus, like stripes on a watermelon (**84**). Scattered rounded lesions are also seen. Portal hypertensive gastropathy may present with a similar appearance, but tends to be more diffuse and less antrum predominant.

The lesions are strings of telangiectatic vessels, which blanch on pressure of biopsy forceps and bleed excessively if biopsied.

Prognosis
The lesions continue to bleed intermittently and chronically in most patients.

Management
A variety of approaches has been tried. Antrectomy is the most radical. Endoscopic therapies include alcohol injection, laser ablation, and argon-plasma coagulation. Corticosteroids and oestrogen–progesterone have also been used. Patients need endoscopic follow-up, as ablated lesions tend to return. Therapy aimed at reducing portal pressure (propranolol, TIPSS) is appropriate for patients with vascular ectasia in association with portal hypertensive gastropathy, but not for those with vascular ectasia without portal hypertension.

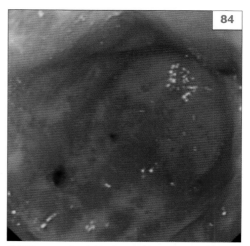

84 'Haemorrhagic' lesions of gastric vascular ectasia. These may produce appearances of 'watermelon' stomach. Argon-plasma coagulation is being used to treat these lesions.

Gastric polyps

Gastric polyps are noted quite frequently as an incidental finding during upper gastrointestinal endoscopy or barium radiology of the stomach.

Definition
'Gastric polyp' is a generic term, which describes a variety of pathologies causing polypoid lesions in the stomach. Histological differentiation is essential.

Epidemiology
Patients usually present in the sixth and seventh decades; males and females are equally affected. Although postmortem studies suggest that gastric polyps are uncommon, they are found in 1–3% of the (selected) population that undergo endoscopy (**85**).

Clinical history
There are no specific symptoms. Frequently, gastric polyps are found incidentally during investigation of unrelated symptoms. Patients can present with dyspepsia, nausea, or weight loss. Anaemia is common, but frank haematemesis is rare. Intermittent gastric outlet obstruction can occur with pedunculated antral lesions.

Pathophysiology
Benign epithelial lesions
Benign gastric epithelial lesions are important because they may, to varying degrees, be premalignant and are potentially curable endoscopically.

Hyperplastic polyps (regenerative polyps)
These are common gastric polyps. They usually occur in the gastric fundus and body as multiple sessile lesions, and have no malignant potential. They are an overgrowth of gastric foveolar and gland tissue. These polyps can be simply excised at endoscopy.

Fundic gland polyps
Fundic gland polyps (**86, 87**) are noted in up to 2% of patients undergoing upper gastrointestinal endoscopy, and are most common in middle-aged women. Typically, they are sessile, less than 5 mm, and occur in the upper stomach. Usually, there are less than 10 polyps but more can be seen. There may be a link with proton pump therapy. The malignant potential of these polyps is very small and endoscopic surveillance is not recommended.

Fundic gland polyposis
This is an association of familial adenomatous polyposis (FAP) and attenuated FAP. Patients can

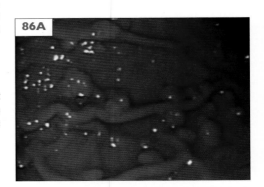

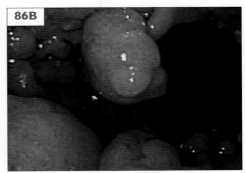

85 An inflammatory polyp seen in the gastric antrum.

86 Multiple gastric polyps seen at endoscopy. Typical cystic glandular polyps are seen in (**A**); occasionally, they can be much larger (**B**).

have their whole stomach studded with polyps (**88**). In FAP, the fundic gland polyps arise due to a mutation in the adenomatous polyposis coli (*APC*) gene. Endoscopic surveillance is warranted, as patients also develop adenomas with the attendant risk of dysplasia and cancer. In the sporadic form of fundic gland polyposis, mutations of the beta catenin gene have been described. Histologically, both forms show dilated cystic fundic glands.

Benign adenomatous gastric polyps
Benign adenomatous gastric polyps arise from gastric glands and tend to occur predominantly in the antrum. Usually, they are solitary, pedunculated, and have tubulovillous architecture. There is a significant risk of malignant change, especially in lesions >2 cm in size. Small lesions can be resected endoscopically, whereas larger lesions require surgery.

Laboratory and special examinations
Endoscopic excision of the whole polyp offers the most certain means of diagnosis. Not all polypoid lesions seen in the stomach are true polyps, and prominent normal folding can be mistaken for a polyp. Patients with polyps seen on barium meal must be referred for endoscopy. Parietal cell and intrinsic factor antibodies, and vitamin B_{12} estimation are indicated to detect pernicious anaemia in patients with adenomas. The large bowel should also be investigated, as there is an association with colonic polyps.

Special polyposis syndromes
Several polyposis syndromes are recognized. Adenomatous polyps are found in the stomach and duodenum of patients with FAP (**88, 89**). The polyps in patients with Peutz–Jehger's syndrome are hamartomas with little malignant potential, but warrant endoscopic removal to reduce the risk of intussusception. In Cronkhite–Canada syndrome (hyperpigment-ation, alopecia, nail dystrophy, and polyposis), polyps are similar to those in Ménétrier's disease.

Management of gastric polyps
The management depends on the histology of the polyp. Small pedunculated polyps can be excised endoscopically, and patients followed up with endoscopic surveillance. In the frail and elderly, this is preferable to surgery with its attendant risks. Patients with rapidly recurring or neoplastic polyps should be offered surgery.

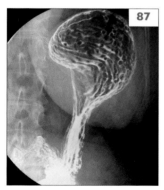

87 Appearance of fundic gland polyps with a barium meal.

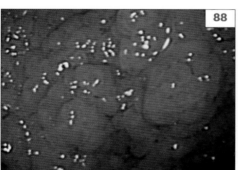

88 FAP – the stomach is carpeted with tiny polyps.

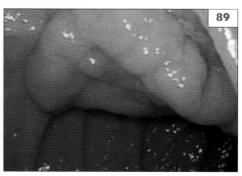

89 Large flat adenoma in the duodenum of a patient with FAP.

Other gastric lesions

GASTROINTESTINAL STROMAL TUMOURS (GISTS)
Definition
GISTs are uncommon tumours that arise from mesenchymal tissue in the gastrointestinal tract, most frequently in the stomach and proximal gastrointestinal tract.

Pathophysiology
GISTs almost always express CD117 antigen (part of a membrane-bound tyrosine kinase, c-kit), and this has assisted classification of these tumours. Current opinion is that they arise from the interstitial cells of Cajal.

Clinical features
GISTs can be detected as incidental findings during investigation of unrelated symptoms, or may present with a palpable mass, pain, or gastrointestinal bleeding. They have a variety of appearances at endoscopy, depending on their location and whether they erode into the lumen of the gastrointestinal tract.

The biological behaviour of GISTs is variable and difficult to predict; larger (>2 cm) lesions and those with a higher mitotic index (a measure of proliferation) are more likely to metastasize.

Management
The principles of management are surgical resection if the lesion is accessible, including resection of metastasis. Imatinib, a specific orally active tyrosine kinase inhibitor, is used for inoperable GIST, and trials of its role in the adjuvant setting are ongoing.

OTHER NONEPITHELIAL LESIONS
Submucosal lipomas can be recognized as they are compressible at endoscopy. Neurogenic and vascular tumours also occur.

Ectopic pancreatic tissue can also occur in the antrum and present as an intramucosal lesion, typically with a central 'dimple' (**90**). Very rarely, intramural gastric duplication cysts cause a smooth indentation in the stomach wall.

Laboratory and special examinations
The diagnosis of nonepithelial lesions is problematic. Endoscopic biopsy may not be adequate for diagnosis in submucosal lesions, and the behaviour of GISTs is difficult to predict. EUS

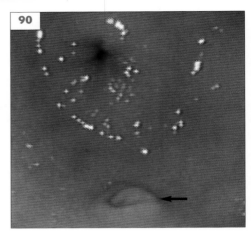

90 Ectopic pancreatic rest seen in the antrum at endoscopy.

with aspiration or core biopsy has proved valuable in diagnosis, and for differentiating submucosal lesions from other causes of extragastric compression.

CT scanning may show the characteristic low-attenuation appearances of lipomas.

Differential diagnosis
Extrinsic compression of the stomach may mimic submucosal tumours or ectopic pancreatic tissue. Gastric lymphoma can be polypoid, and polypoid swelling of rugae occurs in Ménétrier's disease. Carcinoid and amyloid are rare causes of polypoid lesions. Gastric varices due to portal hypertension may appear polypoid and should not be biopsied.

GASTRIC LYMPHOMA
Definition
Gastric lymphoma is a primary gastrointestinal lymphoma of the stomach.

Epidemiology and aetiology
Primary lymphomas of the gastrointestinal tract are rare. The stomach is the most common site, accounting for about half of all cases (**91**).

Peak incidence occurs in the 60-year-old age group, with men affected more frequently than women.

Pathophysiology
Gastric lymphomas present as an ulcer, a diffuse infiltrating lesion, or with giant rugal folds

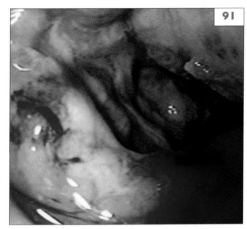

91 Gastroduodenal lymphoma.

Bone marrow examination and thoraco-abdominal imaging are necessary to differentiate this from other extranodal lymphomas.

Differential diagnosis
Gastric lymphoma is frequently misdiagnosed as gastric ulcer. The true diagnosis emerges when the lesion fails to heal. Some are only diagnosed by frozen section from exploratory laparotomy. Several criteria can be used to differentiate a primary gastric lymphoma from a secondary lymphoma spreading from other sites: the absence of palpable lympha-denopathy; no mediastinal lymphadenopathy, and only regional/retroperitoneal lymph node involvement; no hepatic or splenic involvement other than by direct spread; normal bone marrow; and disease confined mainly to the gastrointestinal tract. These criteria no longer pertain in very advanced cases.

Prognosis
The prognosis for gastric lymphoma is better than that for gastric cancer, and 5-year survival rates can exceed 75%. Features associated with good prognosis include: early stage disease; small (<10 cm) size; diffuse histiocytic or large cell histological types; and a good initial response to treatment.

Management
H. pylori eradication can lead to regression of low-grade lymphoma (MALToma) and should be pursued. Close endoscopic follow-up is required. Conventionally, lesions confined to the stomach are treated surgically, while radiotherapy and chemotherapy are used in advanced disease. Rituximab (an anti-CD20 antibody) has been used in patients who relapse.

mimicking Ménétrier's disease. Most gastric lymphomas are B-cell lymphomas. An association between low-grade lymphoma and *H. pylori* has been recognized. There are reports of regression of low-grade lymphoma (MALToma), limited to the mucosa, following eradication of *H. pylori*. This suggests that, in some cases at least, the aberrant lymphocyte proliferation is driven by the presence of the bacterium.

Clinical history
Patients present with nonspecific dyspepsia, anorexia, weight loss, nausea, and vomiting.

Physical examination
An epigastric mass is palpable in 30% of patients.

Laboratory and special investigations
There is commonly anaemia and raised erythrocyte sedimentation rate (ESR). Endoscopic appearances of lymphomatous lesions are similar to those of gastric cancer, but diagnosis is frequently delayed. This is because biopsies are often falsely negative, as the lymphomatous tissue is deep in the mucosa. Multiple snare biopsies are more likely to yield the diagnosis. Radiologically, extension of a lesion from the stomach into the duodenum is suggestive of gastric lymphoma. EUS has a role in evaluating these lesions (depth of invasion, gastric lymph node involvement, guided biopsy) and in assessing response to therapy.

Leiomyomas

Leiomyomas arise in the smooth muscle layers and expand submucosally towards the lumen (**92**). Their apex may ulcerate the mucosa, and lead to presentation with haematemesis. Some leiomyomas also involve the serosal surface of the stomach – 'dumb-bell' tumours. EUS may assist in defining from which mucosal plane the lesion arises. Malignant transformation to leiomyosarcoma may occur.

Duodenum: anatomy and histology

The duodenum passes from the pylorus to the duodenojejunal flexure – a distance of about 30 cm in a normal adult (**93**). There are four parts: the first (the 'duodenal bulb') is 3–5 cm long and is the prime site for duodenal ulcers; the second is 7–10 cm long and receives biliary and pancreatic drainage via the ampulla of Vater; the third and fourth parts complete the duodenal 'loop'. From the ligament of Treitz onwards, the upper small intestine is named the jejunum.

Histology
The histology of the duodenal mucosa is similar to that of the other small-intestinal regions. The intestinal surface of the mucosa and submucosa is thrown into multiple villi, which increase the absorptive area. Specialized epithelial cells are absorptive, with further specialized microvilli on the surface. A unique feature of the duodenum is the presence of Brunner's glands in the submucosal layer (**94**).

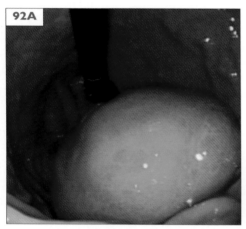

92A

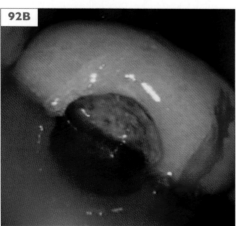

92B

92 An enormous leiomyoma in the stomach (**A**). In (**B**) an area of ulceration and spontaneous necrosis is seen.

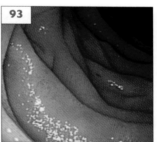

93

93 The normal duodenum seen at endoscopy.

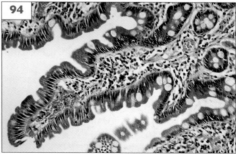

94

94 Normal slim villi of small intestine shown histologically.

Chronic duodenal ulceration

Definition
Chronic ulceration of the duodenum is a common clinical problem and describes the presence of a breach in the duodenal mucosa that has depth. Duodenitis shares a similar aetiology and refers to inflammation in the duodenum. Endoscopically, duodenitis is associated with erosions, which are smaller superficial lesions of the mucosa – an appearance called 'salt and pepper duodenitis'.

Epidemiology
Duodenal ulcers are common in all age groups, but incidence rises with age (by contrast to gastric ulcers, which are rare below 40 years). The lifetime prevalence of duodenal ulceration is about 10% for men and 4% for women, but the prevalence of duodenal ulcers is falling.

Pathophysiology
H. pylori is the most important acquired factor in aetiology and in those not taking NSAIDs; over 95% of duodenal ulcer patients are infected. The mechanism by which antral infection with *H. pylori* results in duodenal ulceration is conjectural. Gastric acid and pepsin are important, and both basal and stimulated gastric acid secretion is higher in duodenal ulcer patients secondary to hypergastrinaemia. This may be attributable to *H. pylori* infection, as may be the apparent familial clustering of duodenal ulcer disease. Alternatively, familial clustering could be linked directly to heritable factors; for instance, blood group O nonsecretor status confers risk. Other factors include cirrhosis, chronic pancreatitis, smoking, and low socioeconomic class. NSAIDs are an important cause of gastroduodenal ulceration.

Clinical history
Patients complain of dyspepsia in relation to food – worsening the pain in some and relieving symptoms in others. Patients complain of many other upper gastrointestinal symptoms and, as with gastric ulcers, these are nondiscriminatory.

Physical examination
Usually, the physical examination is normal. Epigastric tenderness can sometimes be elicited.

Laboratory and special examinations
Barium meal radiology will detect most duodenal ulcers (**95**) and is better than endoscopy for examining the distal duodenum. However, endoscopy is more sensitive, can

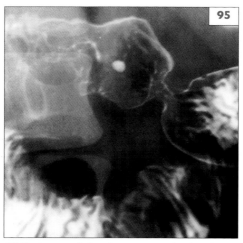

95 Barium meal showing an acute duodenal ulcer as a small round pool of barium.

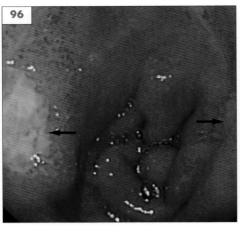

96 Kissing duodenal ulcers.

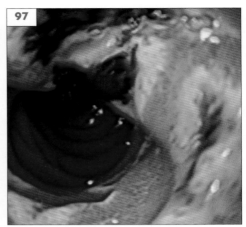

97 Multiple duodenal erosions in a patient taking NSAIDs.

distinguish active ulceration from previous scarring, and can detect very small mucosal lesions. Consequently, it is the preferred mode of investigation (**96, 97**). Antral biopsies can also be taken to diagnose *H. pylori* at the time of endoscopy.

Special forms
Zollinger–Ellison syndrome patients develop multiple duodenal ulcers, secondary to gastrin secretion by tumours. Ulcers can involve the distal duodenum (which is unusual in straightforward peptic ulceration) and some patients have diarrhoea.

Differential diagnosis
Rarely, duodenal ulceration is a manifestation of Crohn's disease, tuberculosis, lymphoma, or sarcoidosis, and, in immunocompromised patients, cytomegalovirus. (In practice, an *H. pylori*-negative duodenal ulcer and lesions distal to the first part of the duodenum should alert the endoscopist to the possibility of these diagnoses.) Pancreatic cancers can erode into the duodenum. Duodenal cancer is very rare.

Prognosis
The natural history of duodenal ulcer disease is relapsing and remitting, unless *H. pylori* is eradicated. Without such eradication, about 80% of patients relapse within a year of healing. Ulcer perforation and bleeding are the most important

complications, and chronic duodenal ulceration can lead to pyloric stenosis.

Management
General management
Smoking impairs ulcer healing and increases relapse, so it should be discouraged. NSAIDs should be discontinued if feasible.

H. pylori eradication
Indications for eradication of *H. pylori* are continually being reviewed, but all infected peptic ulcer patients require *H. pylori* eradication. Remission of symptoms has been advocated as a surrogate marker for eradication. However, in recurrent or complicated ulcers, *H. pylori* eradication should be formally confirmed (e.g. with a urea breath test). Eradication of *H. pylori* reduces the relapse rate to <10% per year. It is likely that the long-term complications of bleeding and perforation will show a similar reduction.

Acid suppression
Duodenal ulcers heal faster than gastric ulcers because they are smaller. Proton pump inhibitors will rapidly heal 90% of duodenal ulcers in 4 weeks. Healing is faster with the more potent acid suppression of proton pump inhibitors compared to H$_2$ receptor antagonists. Resistant ulcers are usually due to smoking, poor compliance, or covert NSAID

and aspirin use. *H. pylori*-associated ulcers will recur on cessation of antisecretory therapy, unless *H. pylori* has been eradicated.

Maintenance acid suppression therapy

Indications for maintenance proton pump inhibitor therapy include: elderly patients (or those with concurrent cardiorespiratory disease), smokers, previous ulcer complication, frequent relapses, severe/protracted symptoms during relapse, and coprescription of NSAIDs in patients with known or previous ulceration. Half the healing dose is given during maintenance. The alternative approach to preventing NSAID ulcer disease is simultaneous use of prostaglandin analogues, but this is frequently limited by side effects.

Surgery

Surgery is indicated for complications, and severe and refractory duodenal ulceration. The highly selective vagotomy is the procedure of choice, as gastric emptying is unimpaired. Former operations included vagotomy and pyloroplasty, vagotomy and gastroenterostomy, and partial gastrectomy (Bilroth II). With the advent of more potent acid suppression with proton pump inhibitor therapy, and eradication of *H. pylori* infection in peptic ulcer patients, elective surgery for duodenal ulceration is now rare.

Complications of peptic ulcers

The most important complications of peptic ulceration (both gastric and duodenal) are gastrointestinal bleeding and perforation. With duodenal ulcers and antropyloric ulceration, there is also the long-term complication of pyloric stenosis, due to scarring and distortion of the pylorus from chronic and recurrent inflammation.

PERFORATION

Typically, patients present with severe and sudden abdominal pain, and lie still with a rigid abdomen. The patient is pale, hypotensive, and very ill. CT scan indicates free intraperitoneal air and, classically, the erect chest radiograph reveals air under the diaphragm (**98**). Perforated peptic ulcer is a surgical emergency. There are reports of conservative management of perforated duodenal ulcers in younger patients but, as yet, this is not routine. Laparotomy is currently the accepted approach.

The operative management of a perforated duodenal ulcer is either simple closure or a definitive procedure to decrease gastric acidity. The experience of the surgeon, the condition of the patient, and the presence of established peritonitis are all factors. Definitive surgery involves closure of the perforation, drainage, and either truncal or highly selective vagotomy.

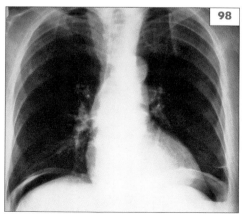

98 Chest X-ray showing 'air under the diaphragm' or pneumoperitoneum, following perforation of a duodenal ulcer.

Perforated gastric ulcers are usually excised at operation because of the risk of malignancy, and reoperation is more frequently required after oversewing a perforated gastric ulcer than a duodenal ulcer. The prognosis is worse in older patients and when peritonitis is more severe.

BLEEDING PEPTIC ULCERS

Bleeding peptic ulcers account for about 50% of acute upper gastrointestinal haemorrhage in the UK. With NSAID and aspirin use, there is a four-fold increased risk of bleeding. Diagnosis is best made by early endoscopy (**99**).

Management

The patient should be resuscitated with blood and colloid.

Pharmacological therapy

This has been disappointing, and no convincing benefit has been demonstrated from acid suppression or antifibrinolytic therapy as initial treatments. There are studies suggesting that high-dose proton pump inhibitor therapy is beneficial for bleeding peptic ulcers, following maximal endoscopic therapy.

Endoscopic treatment

Endoscopic treatment to arrest bleeding from ulcers is now commonly practised. Endoscopic heater probes, laser coagulation, electrocoagulation, endoclips, and injection sclerotherapy are all used. A combined approach using injection therapy (typically dilute epinephrine), followed by a physical method to coapt the bleeding vessel (e.g. application of a heater probe), is probably best. Actively bleeding ulcers, or those with evidence of recent bleeding (for example, adherent clot or pigmented spot in the ulcer base), should receive interventional endoscopic therapy.

Surgery

Normally, 90% of bleeding ulcers stop bleeding with conservative management. The indications for surgery and its timing are controversial. Patients are most successfully managed when there is close liaison between the surgeons and physicians. There should be a low threshold for surgery in an elderly patient with coexistent illness, and a higher threshold for previously fit young patients.

The operation of choice for a bleeding duodenal ulcer is vagotomy and pyloroplasty. Gastric ulcers are managed by Billroth I gastrectomy.

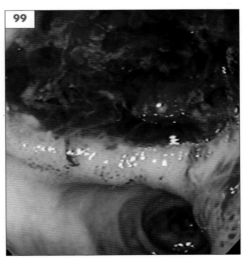

99 Duodenal ulcer with clot in base.

Jejunum and ileum

The diseases predominantly affecting the jejunum and ileum are inflammatory, and tumours are relatively uncommon

Investigation of malabsorption is a pragmatic exercise, based on identifying evidence for malabsorption from blood tests, and securing an anatomical explanation by radiology and biopsy

Immunodeficiency can present with small-intestinal infections

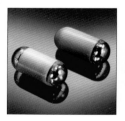 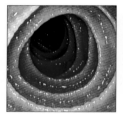 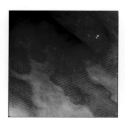 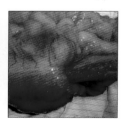

Anatomy and histology

In the normal adult, the small intestine is about 6 m in length, but varies considerably. The change from the jejunum to the ileum occurs at about the halfway point. The jejunum is predominantly in the left upper quadrant; the ileum predominantly in the right lower quadrant, unless malrotation has occurred during foetal development. In about 2% of people, at about 60 cm (2 ft) from the ileocaecal valve, is Meckel's diverticulum. This is a residuum of the developmental umbilical tract, located on the opposite side from that on which the mesentery is attached (antimesenteric border). Meckel's diverticulum is usually 5–8 cm long and may contain ectopic gastric mucosa.

Microscopically, the jejunum and ileum, like the duodenum, demonstrate multiple villi, finger-like protrusions of the mucosa, which increase the absorptive area (**100, 101**).

Investigations of the small intestine

SMALL-BOWEL RADIOLOGY

This may be used to demonstrate anatomy. There are two main techniques (**102, 103**):
- Barium follow-through – ingestion of barium. Small-bowel radiographs are taken as the barium moves spontaneously through the intestine. This is a slow procedure.
- Small-bowel enema (enteroclysis): this involves nasoduodenal or jejunal intubation (under fluoroscopy), followed by rapid infusion of liquid barium. While preferred by some radiologists, patients often find this a difficult procedure.

The appearances of the two techniques differ. In disease, they may show dilatation of the bowel, thickening of bowel wall, strictures, fistulae, and tumours. A technical problem may occur due to barium flocculating in the presence of malabsorption.

Magnetic resonance imaging enteroclysis

As with conventional enteroclysis, there is fluoroscopic intubation of the duodenum. Contrast is introduced, followed by magnetic resonance imaging (MRI) enteroclysis (**104**). Although mucosal detail is not as clear as with conventional enteroclysis, simultaneously examining intra- and extraluminal structures is an advantage. Gadolinium uptake makes it possible to demonstrate areas of active inflammation (e.g. Crohn's disease). Reviewing the images on a computer workstation can also assist in interpretation of areas where loops of bowel overlap, for example.

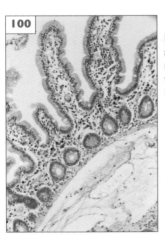

100 Histological appearance of normal villi of the small intestine.

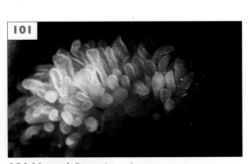

101 Normal dissecting microscope appearance of finger-like villi.

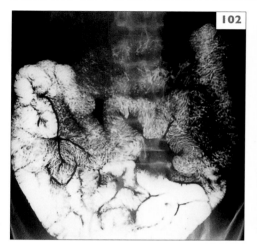

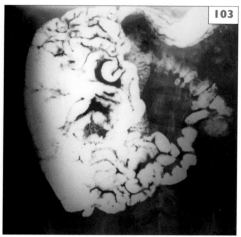

102 Classical small-bowel follow-through appearance, with jejunum at upper right and ileum at lower left of the picture.

103 Malrotation of small bowel identified by small-bowel enema, demonstrating small bowel on the right and caecum to the left.

SMALL-BOWEL ENDOSCOPY
Conventional endoscopy

'Push' enteroscopes, similar in design and principle to conventional upper gastrointestinal endoscopes, extend intubation into the small bowel. 'Push' enteroscopes are longer than normal endoscopes, and usually require an overtube to stabilize them and prevent looping in the stomach. Double balloon enteroscopes use sequential inflation of balloons and an overtube to assist intubation. For both 'push' enteroscopy and double balloon enteroscopy, some estimate of enteroscope position can be made if fluoroscopy is used. As with conventional endoscopy, the enteroscope has an operating channel for biopsy or therapeutic interventions. An alternative technique is 'pull' enteroscopy. In this procedure, an enteroscope passes passively through the small bowel by peristalsis and is slowly withdrawn. Observations are made as the mucosa slips past, and there is no therapeutic capacity.

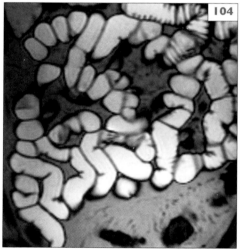

104 Normal small bowel seen with MRI enteroclysis.

Wireless capsule endoscopy (synonym video capsule endoscopy)

An exciting approach to small-bowel imaging has been the development of wireless capsule endoscopy. The capsule is a little bulkier than a large pill, and contains light-emitting diodes (LEDs) as a light source, lens and imager, battery, and antenna (**105–107**). The patient swallows the capsule endoscope. As it is swept through the bowel by peristalsis, the capsule transmits pictures received by sensors in a harness worn by the (ambulatory) patient. Downloaded data are interrogated with software. The views of the small bowel are very clear, and the technique has emerged as an excellent means of visualizing small-intestinal mucosa. It has proved especially valuable in diagnosing small-bowel vascular lesions in patients with obscure or occult gastrointestinal blood loss, as well as in assessing small-intestinal inflammatory and neoplastic disorders.

Jejunal biopsy

Historically, jejunal biopsy was performed using a pneumatic capsule, e.g. Crosby capsule, under fluoroscopy. The method provided a representative sample of mucosa, which was inspected under a dissecting microscope. The convenience of taking duodenal biopsy at endoscopy has replaced this technique for identifying diffuse small-intestinal disease (e.g. coeliac disease).

FURTHER TESTS

Investigations for malabsorption.

Xylose absorption

The 5-hr urinary recovery of orally ingested xylose (nonmetabolized carbohydrate) should be >25%, and is abnormal if the gut mucosa is abnormal. The technique requires normal renal function.

Protein absorption

This is rarely assessed directly.

Fat absorption

In the faecal fat test, after ingestion of 70 g of fat, normally <5 g appears in the faeces in 24 hours. The method requires a 3-day collection period, while ensuring adequate fat intake.

An alternative is the ^{14}C-linoleic acid breath test, which measures fat uptake. Radiolabelled ^{14}C-linoleic acid is given by mouth, and either the serum radioactivity measured, or exhaled $^{14}CO_2$ monitored by a breath test.

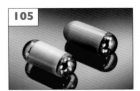

105 The capsules used in wireless capsule endoscopy.

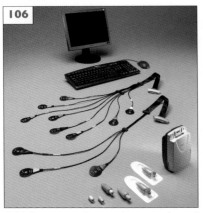

106 Equipment for wireless capsule endoscopy.

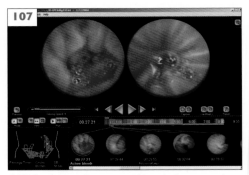

107 Analysis software used in wireless capsule endoscopy.

Investigation of diarrhoea and malabsorption

As discussed in Chapter 1, it is important to define whether a patient is describing changes in consistency, frequency, or volume of stool.

The causes of diarrhoea may be defined physiologically:

- Secretory (e.g. cholera toxin or hormonally mediated neoplastic syndromes) – secretion of salt and water by gut epithelial cells.
- Exudative (e.g. inflammatory bowel disease and ulceration) – loss of interstitial fluid from the inflamed gut wall.
- Osmotic (e.g. ingestion of laxatives such as magnesium salts) – highly osmotic, nonabsorbable substances in the gut lumen prevent water absorption. In malabsorption, nonabsorbed food (e.g. fat) can contribute to osmotic load.
- Hypermotility (e.g. irritable bowel syndrome).

Often, more than one mechanism is present.

INVESTIGATION OF DIARRHOEA

Initially, it is important to elicit a clinical history in order to identify likely causes.

Small-intestinal disease

Here, there is either watery or fatty diarrhoea. Often, there is no pain, and if pain occurs, it is not closely related to defaecation. The presence of blood is unusual. The stool volume may be large.

Pancreatic disease

This is classically steatorrhoea, with pale floating stools, and 'oil on water' from excess fat loss. It may be associated with pancreatic pain after eating (pain in the back, or ill-defined upper abdominal pain).

Colonic causes

This is often associated with colonic pain (lower abdominal colic, below umbilicus, immediately before defaecation, and relieved by passage of stool). The stools are bloody if the condition is associated with inflammation. The stool volume is not large (only 1,200 ml of fluid enters the colon from the terminal ileum daily).

CURRENT APPROACHES

There are two stages. The first is to use the clinical history to localize the probable organ of involvement:

- Small intestine. A positive anti-tissue transglutaminase (tTG) antibody may suggest the diagnosis of coeliac disease – perform duodenal biopsy.
- Pancreas, possibly cancer or pancreatitis – perform ultrasound, CT, magnetic resonance cholangiopancreatography (MRCP), or endoscopic retrograde cholangiopancreatography (ERCP).
- Colonic, possibly neoplasia, diverticular disease, irritable bowel syndrome, colitis – perform sigmoidoscopy/ colonoscopy/barium enema.

Functional tests, i.e. tests of malabsorption, should be needed only if the diagnosis is obscure.

SUSPECTED SPECIFIC MALABSORPTION STATES

Vitamin B_{12}

Vitamin B_{12} absorption is complex and includes:

- Combination of ingested B_{12} with intrinsic factor in the stomach.
- Absorption of intrinsic factor B_{12} complex via specific receptors in the ileum.

In addition, the pancreas is involved in ensuring that the intrinsic factor B_{12} complex is stable. Bacteria in the small intestine may also lead to B_{12} deficiency, due to bacterial utilization of the vitamin.

Vitamin B_{12} deficiency should be suspected if:

- Previous gastric surgery has been performed, especially partial gastrectomy.
- There is ileal disease or resection.
- There is a history of autoimmune disease (leading to gastric atrophy).
- There is vitiligo (autoimmune marker) or peripheral neuropathy.

Blood tests

These include a serum assay for vitamin B_{12}. A high mean corpuscular volume (MCV), and low haemoglobin and low white cell count, reflect B_{12} deficiency (or folate deficiency). Autoantibodies (antiparietal cells, anti-intrinsic factor) indicate the presence of autoimmune disease.

Specific absorption tests

Schilling tests involve ingesting radioactive B_{12}, with simultaneous injection of B_{12} to ensure that binding sites are saturated, and subsequent measurement of absorbed B_{12} by measuring % of B_{12} radioactivity appearing in the urine.

- Part I Schilling test (B_{12} alone) – abnormal in all types of B_{12} malabsorption.
- Part II Schilling test plus intrinsic factor – corrects absorption in gastric abnormality.
- Part III Schilling test (using pancreatic enzymes) – corrects if there is pancreatic deficiency.
- Part IV Schilling test (after antibiotics) – corrects if there is bacterial overgrowth.

LACTOSE AND OTHER CARBOHYDRATES

Upper small-intestinal enterocyte enzymes cause splitting of disaccharides to monosaccharides (e.g. sucrose, split by sucrase, provides glucose–fructose; lactose, split by lactase, provides glucose–galactose; maltose, split by maltase, provides glucose–glucose) prior to digestion. Unabsorbed disaccharides lead to diarrhoea, due to unabsorbed osmotic load, while fermentation in the colon worsens diarrhoea, with excess gas production. Clinically, two forms of deficiency are relevant:

- Genetic lactase deficiency: this is in fact the normal situation, with loss of lactase during development after weaning. About 90% of the world's population lose lactase, in which case ingestion of sufficient milk leads to diarrhoea. Northern European populations tend to maintain the enzyme.
- Acquired lactase deficiency: occurs transiently after small-intestinal infections, or when other diseases (e.g. coeliac disease) lead to loss of enterocyte number and function.

Assessment

Lactose tolerance test

This is a clinical test in which patients drink a solution containing 50 g of lactose. Lactase deficiency is shown by symptoms of diarrhoea developing and by the lack of an increase in blood glucose after 30 mins.

Breath test

Here, 50 g of lactose is ingested. In the absence of lactase, this leads to an increase in breath hydrogen within 2 hr, which reflects the production by gut bacteria of hydrogen from nonabsorbed lactose.

BILE ACIDS

Normally, bile acids are produced in the liver, stored in the gallbladder, and released into the duodenum via the common bile duct after meals. Bile acids facilitate fat by delivering triglycerides to the enterocyte surface (in the form of 'micelles'). Bile acids are reabsorbed in the terminal ileum to return to the liver. There are two degrees of bile acid malabsorption seen after ileal resection:

- Malabsorption with short ileal resection (<1 m). Some bile acids are not reabsorbed and pass into the colon, where they induce colonic secretion. Sufficient bile acid is resynthesized by the liver to maintain normal fat absorption. Treatment is by giving a bile acid-binding agent (cholestyramine) by mouth.
- Larger ileal resection (>1 m). Bile acid loss is such that the liver cannot synthesize sufficient replacement, thus diminishing the bile salt pool. As a result, inadequate bile acids are present in the upper gut, fat absorption is incomplete, and the undigested fat causes steatorrhoea. The large volume of diarrhoea and steatorrhoea is due to colonic fermentation of fat to short-chain fatty acids, which are osmotically active and induce secretion. When bile salts are deficient, there is also a change in the constitution of bile in the gallbladder, and cholesterol gallstones begin to precipitate as cholesterol is not kept in solution. Treatment of steatorrhoea due to bile salt deficiency is by fat restriction. Energy requirements can be satisfied by substituting medium-chain triglyceride oil (or normal dietary fat, although this is often poorly tolerated by patients). These medium-chain triglyceride oils are absorbed directly into portal blood without requiring bile salts.

Abnormal bile salt metabolism can occur for reasons other than ileal disease:

- Liver disease – cholestatic liver disease (obstructive jaundice, primary biliary cirrhosis, etc.) causes decreased bile flow and fat malabsorption.

- Idiopathic bile salt malabsorption also causes chronic persisting diarrhoea. Mutations in the ileal bile acid transporter are reported. Occasionally, idiopathic bile salt malabsorption is unmasked or precipitated by an episode of gastroenteritis. It responds to oral bile sequestration agents (oral cholestyramine).

Differential diagnosis
- Support from history of ileal resection/disease or hepatobiliary disease.
- Bile acid malabsorption can be documented using a radiolabelled synthetic bile acid (SeHCAT). Following an oral dose of SeHCAT, retention is measured after 7 days using a gamma-camera. Less than 10% retention is indicative of bile acid malabsorption.

BACTERIAL OVERGROWTH
Bacterial overgrowth in the common bile duct or upper small intestine can degrade bile acids, impairing fat absorption. Functional testing is by administration of ^{14}C-labelled glycocholic acid, which should be absorbed by the ileum and passed to the liver. If ^{14}C-glycocholic acid is exposed to bacteria (from bacterial overgrowth, or as it is lost into the colon), $^{14}CO_2$ is released, which can be measured in the breath. An early abnormal rise in $^{14}CO_2$ in the breath suggests the presence of bacteria in the upper gut/common bile duct. A late abnormal rise in $^{14}CO_2$ in the breath indicates the passage of excess bile acid to the colon in ileal disease.

Malabsorptive states

Definition
Malabsorption is defined as failure to absorb properly the nutrients present in the gut. It should be distinguished from malnutrition, which is inadequate food intake. However, in malabsorption, patients may appear malnourished.

While absorption is the main function of the small intestine, and malabsorption generally reflects small-intestinal disease, diseases in other organs may also cause malabsorption. For example, the pancreas, in failing to produce digestive enzymes, may cause chronic malabsorption.

Malabsorption may be general for all foodstuffs (for example, diffuse small-intestinal disease), or may be specific (for example, failure to absorb glucose and galactose in milk due to a lack of the enzyme lactase). Generally, the term malabsorption syndrome is limited to patients who have generalized problems with absorption. In such patients, fat malabsorption is generally the biggest problem, so the presence of steatorrhoea – excess fat in the stool – is often taken as the strongest evidence for malabsorption.

Malabsorption can arise for many reasons, which may be classified conceptually.

Conditions in the gut lumen
- Lack of pancreatic enzymes, e.g. chronic pancreatitis.
- Lack of solubilizing bile salts (obstructive jaundice).
- Bacterial overgrowth.
- Inadequate mixing/intestinal hurry (motility disorders, postgastrectomy).

Conditions in the gut wall
- Small-intestinal mucosal disease, e.g. coeliac disease, tropical sprue, Whipple's disease.
- Chronic inflammation, e.g. diffuse Crohn's disease.

Conditions outside the gut wall
- Lymphatic abnormalities, e.g. lymphoma obstructing lymphatic channels.

Inadequate gut length
- Short gut or short bowel syndrome after surgery.

SYMPTOMS AND SIGNS OF MALABSORPTION

Symptoms are highly variable, but diarrhoea, fatigue, and weight loss are common. Signs vary from none to anaemia, pigmentation, finger clubbing (see **2**), and evidence of specific deficiencies – glossitis, cheilosis, hyperkeratosis, night-blindness, purpura, ecchymoses, oedema, and eczema (**108**).

LONG-TERM CONSEQUENCES OF MALABSORPTION

There are a number of physiological problems in other organs following malabsorption. These include:

- Renal stones, which are of two types: (a) oxalate stones, due to excess absorption of dietary oxalate if there is steatorrhoea (with steatorrhoea, there is no free calcium to produce insoluble calcium oxalate that cannot be absorbed); (b) urate stones (from dehydration and a tendency to pass acid urine when diarrhoea is present).
- Osteomalacia: failure to absorb vitamin D, leading to loss of calcium from bone. This is assessed biochemically by low calcium, high phosphate, and increased bony alkaline phosphatase as well as low serum vitamin D. Radiographs may indicate pseudofractures (Looser's zones, **109**), but are less sensitive.
- Night-blindness (vitamin A deficiency).
- Peripheral neuropathy (B_{12} deficiency) in ileal resection only.
- Secondary changes in the pancreas (decrease in digestive enzymes due to malnutrition).
- Gallstones (due to depleted bile salt pool leading to supersaturated bile); these occur with extensive ileal resection.

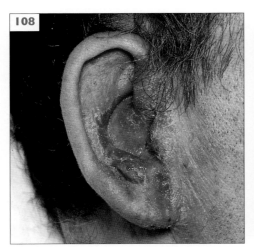

108 Chronic zinc deficiency resulting in chronic eczematous eruption.

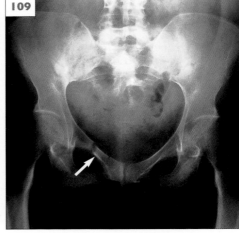

109 Osteomalacia, shown by a Looser's zone, a pseudofracture, clearly seen in the right superior pubic ramus.

Coeliac disease – gluten-sensitive enteropathy

Definition
Coeliac disease is an inflammatory process, which occurs in susceptible individuals in response to the ingestion of wheat protein (gluten and gliadin). The disease affects the small intestine – predominantly the duodenum and jejunum – resulting in changes in small-intestinal architecture, with loss of normal villous architecture and malabsorption of nutrients.

Epidemiology and aetiology
Coeliac disease occurs mainly in people of northern European origin, although it can affect most races. It is most common in Eire, the UK, and northern Europe. Recent studies, where populations have been meticulously screened, show higher prevalence rates than previously appreciated (of the order of 1:300–1:500).

Almost all patients possess the human leukocyte antigen (HLA) haplotype DQ2.5 on chromosome 6. This genetic make-up probably confers the ability to mount a specific immune response to gluten protein in wheat, and can occasionally be useful in establishing the diagnosis.

Pathophysiology
In susceptible individuals, ingestion of wheat results in development of a cell- and antibody-mediated immune response to peptides in wheat gliadin; this response is then expressed in the mucosa of the upper small intestine as wheat is digested. As part of the response, the turnover of epithelial cells of the intestine increases, causing loss of the normal finger-like villi and flattening of the mucosal surface – so-called villous atrophy. The surface area available for digestion falls, and the individual epithelial cells are also abnormal (**110–112**).

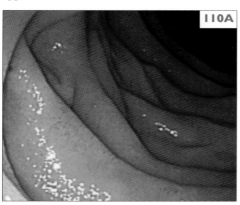

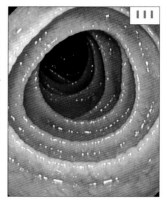

111 Enteroscopy in coeliac disease – scalloped appearance of the mucosal folds is sometimes seen.

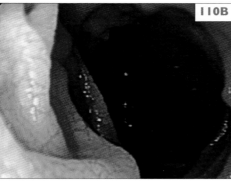

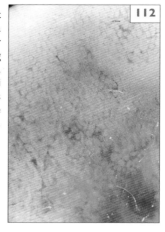

112 Flat jejunal mucosa under dissecting microscope, showing no villi and crypts only (compare with **101**).

110 Endoscopy: (**A**) normal; (**B**) coeliac disease. A subtle 'mosaic' pattern of fissuring in distal duodenal mucosa is sometimes noted in coeliac disease.

Clinical history

This is very variable. In some patients, the condition is manifest as soon as wheat enters the diet, i.e. on weaning, but in others it may not be apparent until late childhood or adult life. Some patients present with a full-blown malabsorption picture – diarrhoea, weight loss, anaemia, and multiple vitamin deficiencies. Others may present with, for example, mild anaemia only, or secondary effects such as infertility or delayed puberty. Some patients are diagnosed on screening family members of a patient – about 10% of first-degree relatives will be affected.

Physical examination

This is also very variable. Often, there are no physical signs. In very severe cases, there may be pigmentation, weight loss, short stature, delayed puberty, anaemia, glossitis, purpura, oedema, and secondary skeletal changes from long-term osteomalacia.

Laboratory and special examinations
Evidence of malabsorption

There are almost invariably low folate levels, low iron, and anaemia. Howell–Jolly bodies seen on the blood film reflect splenic atrophy, which occurs in coeliac disease for unknown reasons. There are also abnormal coagulation tests, low serum albumin, and low serum calcium in severe cases. Serum alkaline phosphatase activity is high if bone disease is present. The conventional diagnostic test is histopathology of the upper small intestine – duodenal biopsy taken at endoscopy (**111**) or (less frequently nowadays) jejunal biopsy (small-intestinal biopsy, 'Crosby capsule', **113**). There are varying degrees of villous atrophy and chronic inflammation, which normalize on gluten withdrawal (**114**).

Blood tests

These are increasingly sensitive and specific and, for some physicians, have replaced biopsy tests in clinical practice. With 'antiendomysial antibodies', the target antigen is tTG, and the tTG ELISA is a sensitive and specific test for coeliac disease. 'Antigliadin' and 'antigluten' antibodies are nonspecific, unless in sophisticated form to detect IgA class antibodies. Antibody titres tend to fall with successful treatment and can be used in monitoring response to gluten withdrawal.

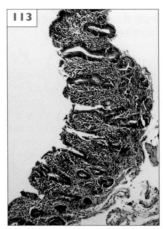

113 Histology of coeliac disease showing flat mucosa and chronic inflammation.

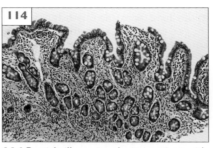

114 Partial villous atrophy in a patient with coeliac disease recovering on a gluten-free diet.

Radiology

Small-intestinal radiographs (small-bowel enema or barium follow-through) may show abnormal mucosal pattern and thickening of jejunal folds (**115**), although these are not specific for coeliac disease. In mild disease, appearances may be normal. In severe, long-standing disease, the changes may be prominent and may also extend into the ileum.

Subtle changes in the small-bowel mucosa of coeliac patients can be detected with wireless capsule endoscopy studies; this may prove useful in detecting complications of coeliac disease.

Special forms

Childhood and adult coeliac disease differ. In childhood, there is a possibility that gluten sensitivity may be transient, and after a time gluten may be reintroduced safely. However, this is rare, even in childhood, and does not seem to occur in the adult.

Occasionally, adult patients do not respond, despite proper dietary therapy (see below). This is loosely called nonresponsive coeliac disease.

Dermatitis herpetiformis
This is a skin condition presenting with a highly itchy eruption on the skin – typically the elbows. Most patients, even if gut symptoms are absent, have a gluten-sensitive enteropathy. Skin and gut improve with withdrawal of gluten from the diet. The condition involves deposition of IgA in the skin.

Differential diagnosis
Coeliac disease should be differentiated from other causes of malabsorption and small-intestinal inflammation:
- In childhood, other food-sensitive enteropathies, i.e. milk sensitivity.
- In adults, Crohn's disease of the small intestine, lymphoma, Whipple's disease.

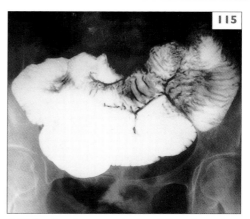

115 Coeliac disease on barium follow-through – note that the valvulae conniventes are thickened and straight in the jejunum.

Prognosis
Treated childhood coeliac disease has an excellent prognosis, provided that dietary treatment is adequate. The gut mucosa returns to normal.

In adults, response may be only partial, with minor continuing histological abnormality, although malabsorption resolves. Long-term complications in adult disease include:
- Small-intestinal lymphoma.
- Development of ulceration of the intestine.
- Small-intestinal cancer.
- Increased incidence of other cancers (e.g. oesophageal cancer).

These complications are discussed below.

Management
Dietary treatment involves the institution of a gluten-free diet. Patient education and dietitian support is vital. Many prepared foods contain unsuspected gluten. A gluten-free diet avoids wheat, wheat products, and rye. Oats and barley are questionable. Rice is permitted.

When disease is very severe, resolution of the intestinal inflammation can be helped by corticosteroids. If response is poor despite strict gluten withdrawal, oral azathioprine may help.

Follow-up
This is important. Checking for early return of deficiencies (Hb, folate, Fe levels) may give early warning of inadequate dietary compliance or complications. Efforts should be made to detect and correct bone loss (osteoporosis and osteomalacia). Evaluation of bone mineral density using dual energy X-ray absorptiometry (DEXA) is usually advocated.

Complications
Complications of coeliac disease include those found at presentation and those that may occur at any time. Those found at presentation are generally the consequences of malabsorption, e.g. anaemia, and are not specific to coeliac disease.

Failure to improve after gluten withdrawal, or relapse after treatment
This is most often due to failure to adhere to the diet – knowingly or unknowingly.

Refractory sprue

This occurs in a minority of patients who fail to respond to a gluten-free diet. Alternative explanations of ongoing diarrhoea to consider are:
- Secondary lactose intolerance (frequently early after diagnosis).
- Bacterial overgrowth.
- Pancreatic exocrine insufficiency.
- Inflammatory bowel disease or microscopic colitis.
- Development of ulcerative ileojejunitis (**116, 117**).
- Development of lymphoma.
- Development of small-intestinal cancer.

Nonspecific ileojejunitis

This is a rare condition, in which ulceration of the jejunum and ileum occurs (nongranulomatous, distinguishing it from Crohn's disease). Symptoms include pain, malabsorption, bleeding, obstruction, and perforation. In some patients, there may be an underlying lymphoma of the small intestine, but this is not always present. Treatment is difficult — both strict gluten withdrawal and corticosteroids are used.

Small-intestinal lymphoma (enteropathy-associated T-cell lymphoma – EATL)

In adults (but not children), 1–3% of individuals will develop lymphoma due to a malignant T-cell clone arising in the small-intestinal mucosa (in contrast to most gut-related lymphomas, which are B-cell associated). Patients present with diarrhoea, weight loss, anaemia, bleeding, or perforation/obstruction. The diagnosis can be difficult to make and laparotomy may be needed to achieve diagnosis. Chemotherapy is generally ineffective and the prognosis is poor. The chances of developing lymphoma fall if patients adhere to a gluten-free diet.

Carcinoma

Adults with coeliac disease have an increased incidence of carcinoma in a number of sites. The risk reduces after gluten withdrawal. Jejunal tumours (presenting with anaemia, obstruction, or frank bleeding) and oesophageal tumours (presenting with dysphagia) are the most common sites.

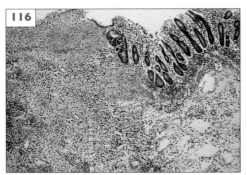

116 Histological section in ulcerative ileojejunitis, showing loss of mucosal epithelium and ulcer formation.

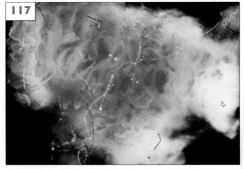

117 Dissecting microscopic appearance in ulcerative ileojejunitis.

Whipple's disease – intestinal lipodystrophy

Definition
Whipple's disease is an infection with the organism *Tropheryma whippelii*, which can affect most organs of the body. It is generally diagnosed when malabsorption occurs, with a characteristic macrophage-rich inflammation of the small-intestinal mucosa (**118, 119**).

Epidemiology and aetiology
This is a rare condition, characteristically but not exclusively affecting middle-aged Caucasian males. The recently described actinomycete, *Tropheryma whippelii* (**120**), can be identified in affected tissues. The mode of transmission and basis of susceptibility is unknown, but the organism can be found in the faeces and in sewage.

Pathophysiology
Affected tissues contain bacteria, and become infiltrated with macrophages. In the intestine, the lymphatics can become blocked, and the normal villous architecture is destroyed, causing malabsorption. Other effects include joint swelling, pleural and pericardial inflammation, and central nervous system (CNS) and meningeal involvement.

Clinical history
Most patients have a history of intermittent arthritis. The diagnosis is usually made when diarrhoea and malabsorption develop. Pleurisy, cardiac involvement (conduction defects, valve problems), and fits and ophthalmoplegia are rare complications.

Physical examination
At diagnosis, pigmentation, clubbing, and other evidences of advanced malabsorption are usually present. Lymphadenopathy, synovial thickening, heart signs, and cranial nerve abnormalities may be present.

Laboratory and special examinations
Diagnosis is most commonly made by examination of small-intestinal histology. A molecular biological approach, using the polymerase chain reaction (PCR) to amplify the bacterial RNA, is needed for identification, as

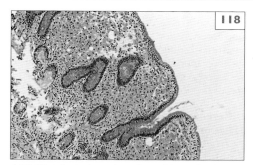

118 Histological section of small intestine in Whipple's disease, with foamy macrophages filling the mucosal space and a lack of normal villous architecture.

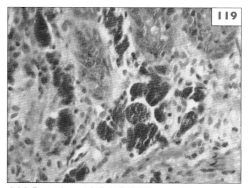

119 Periodic acid–Schiff (PAS) – positive (magenta colour) material characteristic of Whipple's disease in the small-intestinal biopsy.

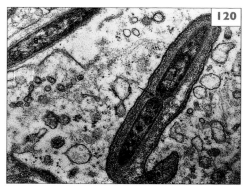

120 Electron microscopic picture showing the Whipple's bacillus – *Tropheryma whippelii*.

the organism is very difficult to culture. Culture is not necessary for clinical management. Small-intestinal radiography shows a characteristic dilated appearance (**121**). Anaemia, folate deficiency, and blood tests indicative of malabsorption will be found.

Differential diagnosis
Differentiate from other causes of malabsorption.

Prognosis
Prognosis is good if the disease is treated early with appropriate antibiotics. Relapsing forms may occur – perhaps indicating the development of antibiotic resistance. CNS and cardiac valve abnormalities do not necessarily reverse after treatment.

Management options
Early and prolonged antibiotic therapy is required. Antibiotics should initially be able to pass the blood–brain barrier, e.g. penicillin and streptomycin, or co-trimoxazole. This is followed by up to a year's oral therapy, e.g. co-trimoxazole, tetracycline.

Short gut or short bowel syndrome

Definition
Short gut or short bowel syndrome (SGS) covers clinical problems arising from reduced intestinal length, following massive intestinal resection (**122**).

Epidemiology and aetiology
In children, the syndrome results generally from surgery for congenital disorders (volvulus, adhesions). In adults, it follows trauma, thrombosis of vessels, Crohn's disease (generally following multiple operations), or ischaemia.

Pathophysiology
The pathophysiology is complex. Two major types may be distinguished:
* Loss of small intestine only.
* Loss of small intestine plus substantial loss of colon.

In the latter group, intestinal problems caused by loss of absorptive capacity are worsened by dehydration due to loss of water-reabsorbing function of the colon.

Short gut syndrome (SGS) generally does not occur if more than half of the length of the small intestine remains. If < 1 m remains, SGS is severe and enteral feeding inadequate. Loss of jejunum

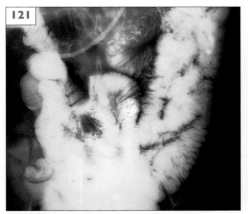

121 Small-bowel enema in a patient with Whipple's disease, showing dilated bowel with thickening of the valvulae conniventes.

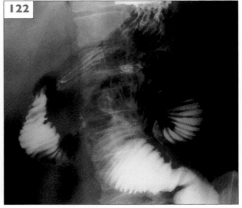

122 Short gut. This barium study shows the stomach, duodenum, 25 cm of jejunum, and distal colon in continuity, after surgery for ischaemia.

is less serious than loss of ileum (the ileum can adapt to take on jejunal functions, but the jejunum cannot take over specific ileal functions such as B_{12} and bile salt absorption).

Malabsorption in SGS is due to:
- Loss of absorbing capacity.
- Presence of undigested fat in intestinal lumen, impairing absorption of other nutrients (e.g. calcium, magnesium).
- Bacterial overgrowth.

Clinical history
The surgical history is obvious, but surgical details are important. Patients with surgically created 'blind loops' in addition to resection are more prone to bacterial overgrowth. Knowledge of the extent of resection and associated colonic loss will define which patients will eventually be able to live without parenteral supplementation, or whether this will be impossible.

Physical examination
Signs of malabsorption, dehydration, and precipitating disease may be present.

Laboratory and special examinations
In SGS, vitamin and mineral deficiencies may develop slowly over years, so magnesium, zinc, copper, selenium, and vitamin A, D, E, and K measurements should be considered. It is useful to document the amount of fat in the stools. Barium follow-through allows measurement of residual intestine, and definition of the presence of strictures and blind loops.

Differential diagnosis
None – although in conditions like Crohn's disease, both disease in the residual small intestine and the lack of length contribute to the severity of the syndrome.

Prognosis
The prognosis is variable. If >1.5 m of small intestine remains, there is a problem in maintaining bodyweight, but it should be possible to maintain near-normal nutrition on a normal diet. If <1 m of small intestine remains, there will be severe problems with malabsorption and weight loss; dehydration will also be a problem if there is ileostomy or substantial

colonic loss. In this group, total parenteral nutrition is often necessary, and this produces its own risk of sepsis and catheter problems.

Management
In the initial stage, parenteral fluid and electrolyte replacement is necessary and, if severe, total parenteral nutrition to prevent excessive weight loss. Some oral feeding is necessary to prevent gut atrophy.

In the subsequent stage, it must be assessed whether adequate fluid and food intake can be maintained orally. Frequent solid food, low lactose and low fat, calorie supplementation with medium-chain triglycerides, and antimotility agents are necessary. If this management is inadequate, total parenteral nutrition will be required.

Complications
Complications are generally related to malabsorption. Renal stones (oxalate, **123**) occur if the colon is intact, due to increased absorption of dietary oxalate. Gallstones occur due to bile salt depletion. Specific vitamin deficiencies include: osteomalacia (vitamin D), night-blindness (vitamin A), and peripheral neuropathy (vitamin E).

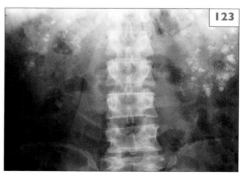

123 Bilateral punctate calcification in both kidneys.

Protein-losing enteropathy

Definition

A variety of gastrointestinal conditions cause protein loss into the gut, leading to weight loss and hypoalbuminaemia. Loss may occur through ulcerated areas, as in inflammatory conditions, or through loss of intestinal lymph, as in lymphangiectasia (**124, 125**). A protein-losing enteropathy (PLE) may be only one aspect of an inflammatory or neoplastic condition affecting the gut, or may be the predominant problem, as in intestinal lymphangiectasia. The causes of PLE are as follows:

- Disorders of the lymphatics – primary lymphangiectasia (familial or sporadic) or secondary intestinal lymphangiectasia (blockage of lymphatic flow by tumour or infection, e.g. tuberculosis, retroperitoneal fibrosis, or inflammation).
- Inflammation and ulcerative conditions – in the stomach, Ménétrier's disease or Zollinger–Ellison syndrome; in the small intestine, coeliac disease, tropical sprue, allergic gastroenteropathy, vasculitis, or Crohn's disease.

Pathophysiology

This varies with the site of protein loss. When loss is from the stomach, symptoms only occur when the liver cannot increase albumin synthesis sufficiently to maintain plasma oncotic pressure, so oedema occurs. In these circumstances, absorption from the small intestine is normal and nutrition is generally maintained. In small-intestinal lymphangiectasia, loss of fluid from

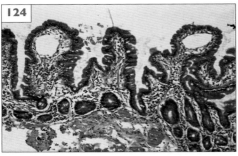

124 Intestinal biopsy showing lymphangiectasia – dilated lymphatic spaces at the tips of the villi.

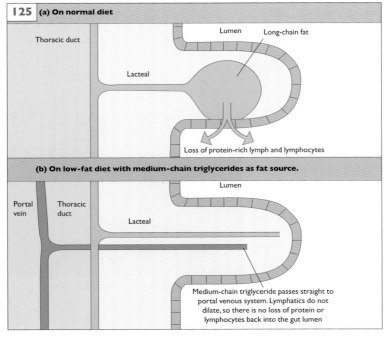

125 (a) On normal diet

Thoracic duct

Lacteal

Lumen   Long-chain fat

Loss of protein-rich lymph and lymphocytes

(b) On low-fat diet with medium-chain triglycerides as fat source.

Portal vein   Thoracic duct

Lacteal

Lumen

Medium-chain triglyceride passes straight to portal venous system. Lymphatics do not dilate, so there is no loss of protein or lymphocytes back into the gut lumen

125 Mechanism of protein loss in lymphangiectasia.

dilated lymphatic channels (lacteals) leads to hypoalbuminaemia, hypogammaglobulinaemia, and leakage of long-chain fatty acids as the dilated lymphatics rupture into the intestine (**126–128**). Lymphocyte loss (T-cells) also occurs. Patients develop steatorrhoea and diarrhoea, and are susceptible to infections.

Clinical history
Symptoms are:
- Characteristic of primary cause (e.g. pain and diarrhoea with Crohn's disease, anorexia and weight loss with gastric cancer).
- Oedema caused by low plasma proteins.
- Malabsorption (if part of intestinal lymphangiectasia).

Physical signs
Oedema and other evidence of malabsorption are present. In intestinal lymphangiectasia, there may be other lymphatic abnormalities, such as long-standing peripheral lymphoedema.

Laboratory examinations
Hypoalbuminaemia and hypogammaglobulinaemia occur, in the absence of liver disease or renal loss. In intestinal lymphangiectasia, there is a low circulating lymphocyte count. To prove the extent of PLE, dynamic tests are required to document the loss of an intravenously injected isotope (i.e. ^{51}Cr-labelled albumin), based on faecal collection.

An alternative nonisotopic method is to measure the clearance of alpha-1 antitrypsin from stool and plasma measurements. Alpha-1 antitrypsin leaked into the gut resists proteolysis and intraluminal degradation, and is stable to measure in the stool.

Anatomical studies are required to identify the nature and site of protein loss. Endoscopy and barium meal will demonstrate lesions in the stomach (thickened folds of Ménétrier's disease, gastric lymphoma, or hypersecretory syndromes). Small-intestinal radiograph studies may show:
- Generalized oedema reflecting hypoproteinaemia.
- Characteristic signs of lymphoedema.

Differential diagnosis
PLE is generally part of another syndrome. In intestinal lymphoma, differential diagnosis is between the primary and secondary causes. CT scanning will exclude mesenteric or

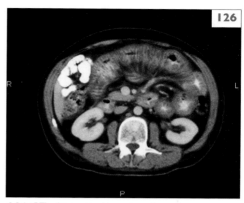

126 CT of intestinal lymphangiectasia.

127 Patients with lymphangiectasia frequently have peripheral lymphatic abnormalities leading to asymmetrical oedema of the legs.

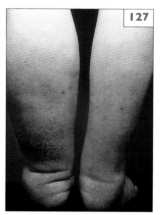

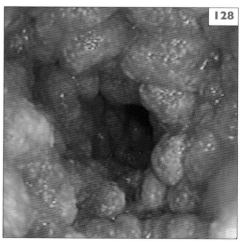

128 Endoscopic appearance of lymphangiectasia.

retroperitoneal lymphadenopathy (126). Peripheral lymphoangiography will identify peripheral lymphatic abnormalities.

Prognosis

If part of an associated condition, then prognosis of that condition should be considered. Primary lymphangiectasia presenting in childhood may be very severe, and even with dietary management, patients may remain with malabsorption and be prone to infection.

Management

If part of an associated condition, then management of that condition should be considered. In Ménétrier's disease, anti-inflammatory drugs have been tried with little effect; in severe cases, gastrectomy has been used. In small-intestinal lymphangiectasia, disease is occasionally limited to small segments, so surgery can be performed, but this is infrequent. If not, dietary treatment is the main approach, in particular a strict low-fat diet, with medium-chain triglycerides to provide calories (this form of fat does not pass through lacteals, see **125**), and identification and treatment of nutrient deficiencies.

Tropical sprue; postinfectious malabsorption

Definition

This is acute or chronic diarrhoea and malabsorption, occurring in the developing world, and associated with abnormal small-intestinal mucosal structure. It is probably attributable to infection. Two forms are distinguished – acute and chronic.

Epidemiology and aetiology

Acute epidemics of sprue affecting whole villages are reported in Asia, probably following acute infections. Chronic tropical sprue was most often recognized in expatriates living in developing countries. Viral infections may initiate acute sprue, while bacterial infection may be responsible for chronic sprue. The distinction between the two forms is not absolute, and traveller's malabsorption seen, for example, in overland hikers returning from Asia may be part of the same spectrum.

Pathophysiology

There are abnormalities in the small-intestinal mucosa leading to malabsorption. Severe folate deficiency may prevent the mucosa from undergoing its normal proliferative cycle.

Clinical history

Acute sprue describes the emergence of prolonged diarrhoea, with varying degrees of malabsorption, after an acute diarrhoeal illness. Chronic sprue may present insidiously with diarrhoea, weight loss, and anaemia, sometimes after returning to a temperate climate.

Physical examination

Signs of malabsorption and weight loss may be present.

Laboratory and special examinations

Attempts must be made by routine techniques to culture single pathogens. There may be laboratory evidence of malabsorption and resulting deficiencies. Anaemia, macrocytosis, and folate deficiency are generally present.

The most specific test is small-intestinal biopsy, which shows abnormal villous architecture, with varying degrees of flattening of the villous pattern (rarely as severe as in coeliac disease). It is important to realize that any dweller in the tropics may have deviations from the normal Western-type villous pattern of finger-like mucosal projections, and minor abnormalities and predominantly leaf-like villi may be the norm (**129**).

Differential diagnosis

The disease must be differentiated from other malabsorptive states such as coeliac disease, and from single-agent infections such as giardiasis. Persistent diarrhoea with no evidence of malabsorption after acute gastroenteritis may merely be postinfectious irritable bowel.

Management options and prognosis

Antibiotic therapy (e.g. tetracycline for 2 weeks) plus folic acid replacement (for some months) is recommended. In severe cases, replacement of other deficiencies may be required. Parasitic infestation such as giardiasis may require specific antimicrobial treatment (e.g. metronidazole).

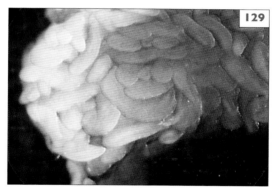

129 Dissecting microscopic appearance showing leaf-like villi (compare with 101).

Bacterial overgrowth

Definition

Bacterial overgrowth is defined as bacterial colonization of the small intestine, leading to malabsorption of one or more nutrients.

Aetiology and epidemiology

This is an uncommon condition, which occurs in the presence of: (a) anatomical abnormality in the small intestine; or (b) rarely, functional abnormality of immune defence.

The anatomical predisposing causes are:
- Jejunal diverticulosis (**130**).
- Previous surgery causing blind loops.
- Crohn's disease when subacute obstruction or enteroenteric fistulae are present.
- Pseudo-obstruction due to motility disorders.
- Infiltration or degenerative disorders affecting motility (e.g. systemic sclerosis, **131**; amyloidosis).

Functional causes include:
- Loss of gastric acidity (pernicious anaemia, long-term acid-suppressive therapy), which removes the generalized first line of defence against ingested bacteria.
- Immunodeficiency syndrome (e.g. hypogammaglobulinaemia, HIV).

Pathophysiology

The upper small intestine is normally sterile, except for transient passage of ingested bacteria. Colonization occurs when 10^6/ml or more bacteria are found on duodenal or small-intestinal aspiration. Bacteria cause diarrhoea in a number of ways:
- Bile salt deconjugation leads to fat malabsorption.
- Nutrient uptake by bacteria leads to deficiencies (e.g. vitamin B_{12} deficiency) and, rarely, hypoproteinaemia, following loss of essential amino acids.

Occasionally, as in a patient with a jejuno-ileal bypass for morbid obesity, in whom a large blind loop (the majority of the small intestine) is present, an immune response to the bacteria can induce systemic symptoms of arthritis and skin lesions (**132**).

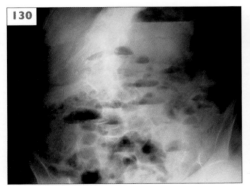

130 Multiple jejunal diverticula containing fluid levels on a plain X-ray, in a patient with bacterial overgrowth.

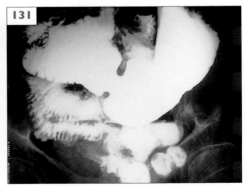

131 Barium meal and follow-through in a patient with systemic sclerosis, showing dilated hypomotile intestine, a breeding ground for bacterial overgrowth.

Clinical history
Episodes of diarrhoea, or chronic diarrhoea; history of a response to antibiotics is often helpful.

Laboratory and special examinations
To establish a diagnosis of bacterial overgrowth, it is desirable to demonstrate:
- The cause (generally anatomical).
- The presence of bacteria.
- A response to antibiotics.

Difficulties in satisfying these criteria may arise because the techniques for demonstrating the presence of bacteria are not satisfactory, because culture of bacteria is difficult to achieve, or because recolonization takes place rapidly after treatment.

To demonstrate the cause, use a barium follow-through. To demonstrate the presence of bacteria, use:
- Functional tests – breath hydrogen test, ^{14}C-glycocholic acid breath test (**133**).
- Urinary indicans (bacterial metabolites).
- Direct intubation, counting, and culture (this needs full bacteriological facilities, particularly for culture of anaerobes).

Special tests
Occasionally, sophisticated tests of gastrointestinal immune system (measuring IgA levels in blood and IgA cells in mucosa) may be needed.

Differential diagnosis
Differentiate from other malabsorption syndromes.

Prognosis
Generally, bacterial overgrowth of the small intestine is not a severe condition, unless it has been unrecognized for a long time and complications such as peripheral neuropathy, due to B_{12} deficiency, have occurred.

Management
Occasionally, blind loops may require surgical correction. More often, intermittent courses of antibiotics are helpful, although repeated episodes of antibiotic treatment may be needed. Empirical regimes include short courses of:
- Tetracyclines.
- Metronidazole.
- Ciprofloxacin.
- Erythromycin.

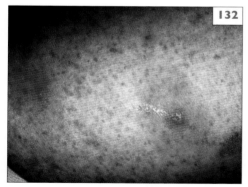

132 Part of the 'arthritis dermatitis' syndrome seen in a patient with jejuno-ileal bypass. This is probably an immune reaction to bacterial overgrowth.

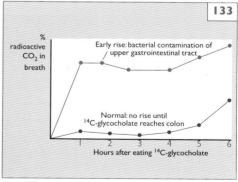

133 ^{14}C-glycocholic acid breath test to detect bacterial overgrowth.

Radiation enteritis

Definition
Radiation enteritis involves inflammation of the intestine as a result of therapeutic irradiation. Acute radiation enteritis occurs at the time of radiation, but chronic damage may occur from months to many years afterwards.

Aetiology, epidemiology, and diagnosis
This is generally seen in middle-aged and elderly females (after radiation of carcinoma of the cervix and uterus), or in elderly males (carcinoma of the prostate). It is more likely to occur with:
- High doses of radiation.
- Radiation after previous surgery (adhesions lead to fixed bowel in the radiation field).
- Genetic susceptibility.

Irradiation leads to chromosomal breakage, cell death, secondary fibrosis, and vasculitis.

Pathophysiology
In acute radiation enteritis, loss of mucosal cells and enhanced motility contribute to diarrhoea. In chronic cases, fibrosis (**134**) and local ischaemia secondary to vasculitis lead to mucosal damage, structuring, and/or fistula formation.

Clinical history
In acute radiation enteritis, nausea and diarrhoea occur during, and for some weeks after, irradiation. Diarrhoea may be fairly severe, but is generally mild and well tolerated. Chronic radiation enteritis affecting the colon presents with diarrhoea, pain, and bleeding. Symptoms are diarrhoea, pain, and malabsorption when the small intestine is involved. Symptoms may be delayed for up to 20 years postirradiation. In association, radiation cystitis may occur with frequent urinary tract infections.

Physical examination
Generally, there are cutaneous signs of irradiation (pigmentation and telangiectasia) in the abdominal field. Weight loss and signs of malabsorption may be seen.

Laboratory and special examinations
Acute radiation enteritis is generally self-limited and needs no investigation. The predominant aim of investigation in chronic enteritis is to define the severity and extent of radiation damage. For small-intestinal disease, radiographic examination (intubated enema or barium follow-through) can be used to define narrowing and structuring, and

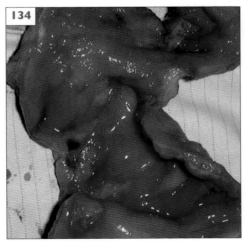

134 Resection specimen of radiation enteritis showing ulceration and thickening of the bowel wall.

irregularity in mucosa. CT scans and MR imaging also help investigate fistulae. Serum B_{12} levels are generally low after pelvic irradiation, due to damage to the terminal ileum. For suspected colonic damage, barium enema and colonoscopy should be used; the prime site is the rectosigmoid, so limited investigation is often all that is needed. Irradiated tissue may be friable; biopsy is diagnostic when histology shows fibroblast proliferation and vasculitis.

Differential diagnosis
The most important differential diagnosis is local recurrence of the original cancer (see also 'Radiation colitis', Chapter 8).

Management
Acute radiation enteritis is managed expectantly; management of chronic radiation enteritis may be very difficult. There is no specific medical treatment for small-intestinal radiation enteritis, other than management of diarrhoea and malabsorption with antimotility agents, replacement of nutrient deficiencies, and, if severe steatorrhoea is present, the introduction of a low-fat diet. Mild colitis may improve with local corticosteroids and 5-amino-salicylic acid (5-ASA) as for ulcerative colitis, but these are often not effective. With narrowing of the gut lumen by fibrous stricture, a low-residue diet may help. Surgery requires great care. Resectional surgery can be performed for local disease – the main consideration is to ensure that two ends of the bowel with residual irradiation damage are not reanastomosed.

Crohn's disease

Definition
Crohn's disease is a chronic and relapsing inflammatory disease of unknown aetiology. Any part of the intestine can be affected, although distal ileal, ileocaecal, and colonic are the most common distributions. Inflammation can extend through all areas of the gut wall, and about 60% of cases include granulomatous inflammation (**135, 136**).

Aetiology and epidemiology
Crohn's disease is more common in northern Europe and North America than in southern Europe or developing countries. It commences at any age, but peaks in teenagers to 30-year-olds,

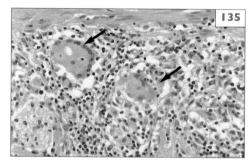

135 One characteristic histological feature of Crohn's disease is granulomas. This plate shows two large giant cells in the submucosa in a patient with Crohn's disease.

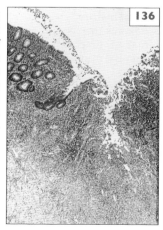

136 A second pathological feature of Crohn's disease is deep fissuring ulcers and inflammation as seen here.

followed by a late peak in the elderly. Unlike ulcerative colitis, the incidence of Crohn's disease is increasing. The aetiology is unknown. Most evidence favours abnormal immune responses – overexpression of inflammatory responses against antigens (bacteria, viruses, food, or autoantigens) in the gastrointestinal tract. Other theories include specific infectious agents (candidates include atypical *Mycobacterium* and measles), but there is no agreement. Smoking is more common in Crohn's disease patients and seems to promote the disease, suggesting environmental influences on aetiopathogenesis. In 15–20% of cases, there will be a family history. A genetic contribution to the disorder is also clear from twin studies. Recently, potential susceptibility genes have been proposed, including genes influencing immune recognition and response to bacterial cell wall components.

Pathophysiology

Inflammation of the gut in Crohn's disease leads to oedema, mucosal thickening, surface ulceration, and often fibrosis of gut wall. In the small intestine, these processes can lead to diarrhoea (due to malabsorption, particularly if bile acid malabsorption occurs in the terminal ileum), pain (from the inflamed bowel irritating the peritoneum and from obstruction to the passage of luminal contents due to oedema and fibrosis), and weight loss. In the colon, inflammation causes exudative bloody diarrhoea. Systemic reactions to the inflammation lead to extraintestinal manifestations affecting joints, skin, and eye.

Clinical history

Symptoms may be present for a considerable period of time, typically 3–4 years, before diagnosis is made. The symptoms depend on the distribution of the disease. Crohn's disease can affect any part of the gastrointestinal tract, although the most common pattern is: terminal ileal disease (one-third of patients), ileocaecal disease (40–50% of patients), and colonic (20% of patients).

Nonspecific symptoms include malaise and weight loss. Extraintestinal symptoms (presenting at some time in 25–35% of cases) include arthritis (small and medium-sized joints), spondylitis, iritis, conjunctivitis, skin lesions (erythema nodosum and pyoderma gangrenosum), and aphthous ulceration of the mouth.

Gastric Crohn's disease

This is generally found coincidentally on biopsy (15% of cases) in adults (**137**).

Duodenal Crohn's disease

This may mimic peptic ulceration and be prone to stenosis or, very rarely, bleeding. Surgery may include strictuloplasty or bypass with gastroenterostomy (**138, 139**).

Small-intestinal Crohn's disease

Diffuse jejunal Crohn's disease is uncommon and can present with weight loss, iron deficiency, hypocalcaemia, and PLE. Disease in the distal ileum or ileocaecal is the commonest location. This usually presents with colicky pain, diarrhoea, abdominal tenderness (particularly in the right iliac fossa as the terminal ileum area is most often involved), and weight loss. With time, Crohn's disease of the terminal ileum leads to narrowing of the small intestine, and repeated episodes of subacute obstruction. This symptom can reflect either a fibrous stricture or active inflammation; deciding which is a common clinical problem.

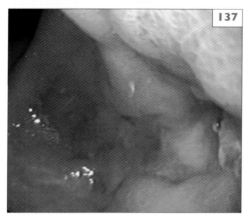

137 Endoscopic appearance of gastric ulcer due to Crohn's disease.

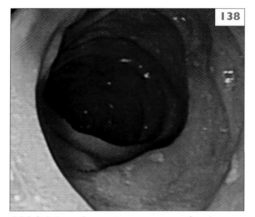

138 Subtle endoscopic appearance of early or mild Crohn's disease as multiple aphthoid ulcers in the distal duodenum.

139 Crohn's disease in the second part of the duodenum, here seen on a barium study.

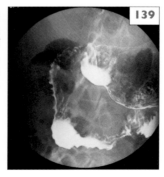

If surgery is performed (see below), removing the affected area of terminal ileum, there is a 50% chance that symptomatic inflammation will return over 5 years (often less) and that repeat surgery will be needed in about 10 years (**140–146**).

Colonic Crohn's disease

Colonic Crohn's disease presents with diarrhoea, either bloody or watery, but often similar to that in ulcerative colitis. It is managed in a similar way to ulcerative colitis, and surgical resection may be required.

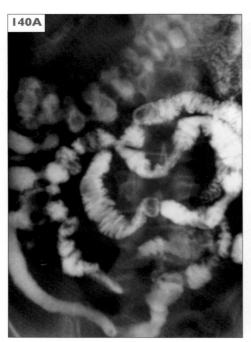
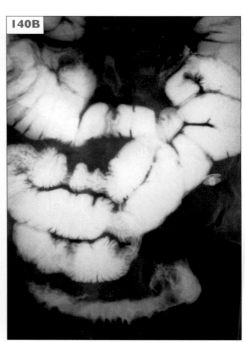

140 Two examples of Crohn's ileitis seen with small-bowel follow-through: (A) showing the increased distance between the loops of bowel; and (B) the 'rose-thorn' ulcers.

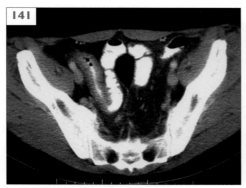
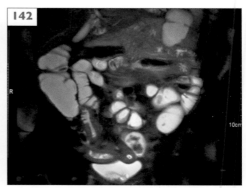

141 Crohn's ileitis seen with CT – note thickening of distal ileal mucosa.

142 Crohn's ileitis seen with MR enteroclysis – note the loops of thickened bowel wall.

Perianal Crohn's disease

Up to one-third of Crohn's patients will have perianal problems (fistulae, abscesses) at some time.

The management of low perianal fistulae (internal openings below the internal anal sphincter) is relatively straightforward – treatment of local infection, discharge, and pain. High perianal fistulae are more problematic, particularly if overtreated surgically, as they may destroy the anal sphincter mechanism.

The principles of treating perianal Crohn's disease are:

- Control local infection. Perianal fistulae may respond to antibiotics – particularly metronidazole or ciprofloxacin.
- Surgical 'toilet' – involving probing under anaesthesia, with incision of abscesses and conservative exploration to maintain drainage. This may be required for severe or recurrent disease, or if there is association with abscess formation.
- Drainage of infection to prevent abscess formation, which may require placement of setons.
- Control of concurrent colonic Crohn's disease with medical therapy.
- Infliximab or other anti-TNF strategies (see 'management options').

In severe perianal Crohn's disease, proctectomy may be indicated.

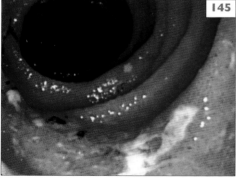

143 Wireless capsule endoscopic appearance of Crohn's disease in the small intestine.

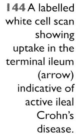
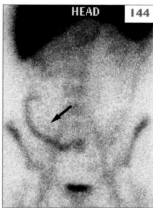

144 A labelled white cell scan showing uptake in the terminal ileum (arrow) indicative of active ileal Crohn's disease.

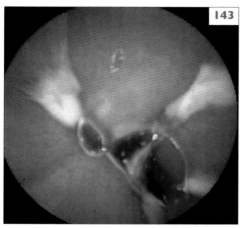

145 Ileocolonoscopy – active Crohn's in the terminal ileum.

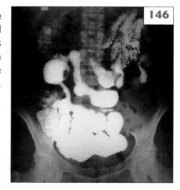

146 Diffuse small-bowel Crohn's disease with multiple strictures.

Fistulae

These can occur between different parts of the gut (ileoileal, ileocolonic, gastrocolic), between the gut and other organs (bladder), or between the skin and gut (enterocutaneous fistulae).

Ileoileal fistulae may be asymptomatic, but predispose to bacterial overgrowth. Ileovesical fistulae cause urinary infection and pneumaturia. Gastrocolic fistulae cause vomiting, severe diarrhoea, and weight loss.

Fistulae are difficult to identify at endoscopy (**150**) but can be seen with barium radiology (**151**).

Abscesses

These may develop locally from the gut, through fissures in the diseased gut wall. Like fistulae, they most commonly occur above areas of stenosis. Free perforation rarely occurs. Abscesses may be a cause of high fever and discomfort. The differential diagnosis is usually from active inflammation in the bowel wall, although the two can also coexist.

Physical examination

Often, there are no abnormalities on examination. Possible findings include anaemia, spondylitis,

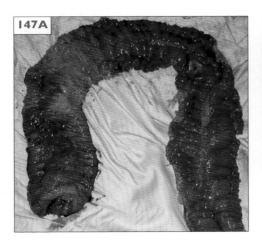

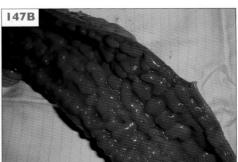

147 Crohn's colitis. Note the patchy distribution of the lesions in this resection specimen (**A**) and, in magnified view (**B**), the oedematous 'cobblestone' mucosa.

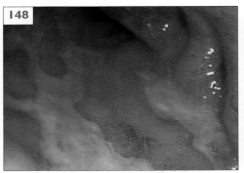

148 Deep serpiginous ulcers seen at colonoscopy in Crohn's colitis.

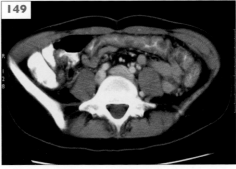

149 Oedematous transverse colon in a patient with fulminant Crohn's colitis.

pigmentation, clubbing, perianal abscesses and fistulae, abdominal masses, and cutaneous fistulae.

There may be stomas or scars commensurate with previous surgery.

Investigations

The spectrum of radiological, histological, endoscopic, and general studies should be tailored to the distribution of the disease (**147–152**).

General studies

- Full blood count, profile.
- To identify inflammation – ESR, C-reactive protein (CRP), low serum albumin.
- To identify deficiencies – B_{12} (notably in terminal ileal disease), folate, iron. If weight loss exists, malabsorption screening may be indicated. Severe malabsorption suggests diffuse jejunal disease (5% of patients).

Special investigations

These will depend on clinical suspicion of the disease distribution, and local availability of the different modalities.

Suspected gastroduodenal disease

Upper gastrointestinal endoscopy or barium studies (**138–139**) should be used.

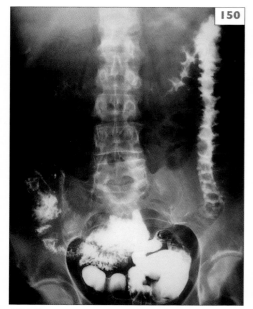

150 Extensive involvement of the descending colon with deep 'rose-thorn' ulcers in Crohn's disease.

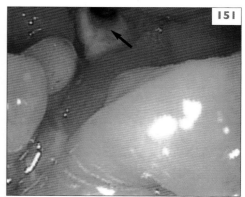

151 Enteroenteric fistulae can be hard to identify at endoscopy. This picture shows the site of an enterocolic fistula (arrow).

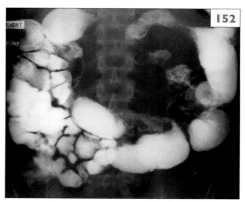

152 A series of different enteroenteric fistulae illustrated with barium study.

Suspected terminal ileal disease or ileocaecal disease

- Radiology – small-bowel studies, either small-bowel enema, follow-through, or MR enteroclysis (**140–142, 146**).
- Wireless capsule endoscopy – detects subtle mucosal disease beyond the resolution of conventional barium contrast radiology (**143**).
- Endoscopy – colonoscopy with terminal ileum intubation and biopsy (**145**).

Suspected colonic disease

Barium enema, colonoscopy (**148**), and biopsy are appropriate. CT is sometimes used (**149**), especially in acute colitis where there are concerns regarding the use of barium studies or colonoscopy. 'Cross-sectional' radiology with CT scanning is also appropriate, particularly if inflammatory abscesses are being assessed. MR imaging identifies bowel-thickening abscesses and fistulae.

Additional techniques

- White cell scanning – identifies areas of inflammation (**144**).
- Ultrasound – can identify thickening of the bowel wall.

Differential diagnosis

Differential diagnosis of Crohn's disease varies, depending on the major sites involved:

- Colonic Crohn's disease – ulcerative colitis, colonic or metastatic cancer, ischaemic colitis in the elderly.
- Ileocaecal Crohn's disease – tuberculosis, intestinal lymphoma. Chronic appendix abscess.
- Acute onset terminal ileal disease – *Yersinia* infection.
- Drugs (potassium chloride, nonsteroidals) – may cause gut ulceration.

Other differential diagnoses include alternative causes of malabsorption (coeliac disease) and gastrointestinal manifestations of immuno-deficiency.

Prognosis

Crohn's disease is currently regarded as 'a disease for life'. The vast majority of patients have normal life expectancy, although some excess mortality due to severe disease and surgical complications occurs, particularly with complex fistulating disease. After surgery to remove disease, recurrence is usual after a mean of 5–10 years, especially in cigarette smokers. In colonic Crohn's disease, there is a small but definite increase in the risk of colonic cancer.

Complications

Urinary problems in Crohn's disease include enterovesical fissure, or right hydronephrosis due to ileal obstruction.

Renal disease may occur if amyloidosis develops. In the presence of marked steatorrhoea, oxalate stones may form in the renal tract.

Gallbladder complications include gallstones (common, due to ileal disease and depletion of bile salt pool) and B_{12} deficiency (due to loss of B_{12} uptake sites, which are limited to terminal ileum).

Management options

- Patient education; doctor/patient empathy (long-term follow-up is very important).
- A team approach with gastrointestinal radiologists, specialist nurses, dietitians, and gastrointestinal physicians and surgeons is required.
- Smoking cessation advice – recurrent disease is more frequent in active smokers.
- Nutritional support.

Medical management

Acute management

This is required for active inflammatory disease (high ESR, CRP), and depends on the predominant site of disease:

- For small-intestinal disease – oral prednisolone (usually for several months). There is some additional benefit from 5-ASA (mesalazine).
- For colonic Crohn's disease – prednisolone (locally for distal disease, orally for pancolitis), and sulfasalazine or mesalazine.

Long-term treatment

Maintaining remission is problematic. There is limited evidence for efficacy of 5-ASA drugs. Some patients require long-term immunosuppressants (i.e. azathioprine, 6-mercaptopurine, methotrexate) to control inflammation. Long-term corticosteroid therapy should preferably be avoided. New 'poorly absorbed' (and rapidly metabolized) steroids (e.g. budesonide) are now available, but are unlikely to be used for long-term therapy.

The cytokine TNFalpha has emerged as a key therapeutic target to modify the inflammatory activity in inflammatory bowel diseases. Drugs derived from antibodies to TNFalpha, such as infliximab and adalimumab, are used in patients with fistulous perianal Crohn's disease or active luminal Crohn's disease, refractory to other therapy.

Some dietary approaches (e.g. elemental diets) help to induce remission, especially in children with small-bowel disease.

Surgical management
Indications for surgery include failure to respond to medical treatment, chronic continuous disease, obstruction with fistulae, and abscess. The most common indication for surgery is recurrent subacute obstruction due to fibrotic terminal ileal stenosis. About 70% of patients will come to surgery at some time.

Ileostomies

Definition
Ileostomies result from surgical operation, the procedure resulting in opening of the ileum through the anterior abdominal wall.

Characteristics
There are two types of ileostomy:
- Temporary ileostomies: performed as an interim stage when multistage colonic surgery is being performed.
- Permanent or 'spout ileostomies' (**153**): these are the most common type, and are used after removal of the colon (for ulcerative colitis or Crohn's disease). 'Continent' ileostomies (e.g. Koch's ileostomy) produce a pouch of ileum below the abdominal wall, which is then drained intermittently via a catheter.

Permanent ileostomies are less common nowadays after total colectomy for ulcerative colitis or familial polyposis, as these conditions are more usually treated by the creation of an ileoanal pouch.

Complications
- Local excoriation of skin and stoma.
- Subacute obstruction of distal ileum proximal to stoma.
- Excessive fluid loss and dehydration in hot weather.
- Urinary tract stone formation (urate stones) due to passage of concentrated acid urine, reflecting loss of alkali and fluid via ileostomy.
- Psychological problems. Support from fellow patients and stoma nurses is very helpful.

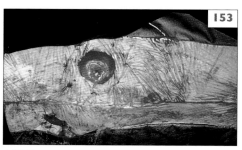

153 Ileostomy.

Immunodeficiency states

Definition
Immunodeficiency states are clinical syndromes reflecting loss of gastrointestinal immune function. The gastrointestinal disease generally results from inability to control infection.

Aetiology and epidemiology
This is very varied. The condition may be genetic or acquired, and may affect different arms of the immune system. Loss of antibodies occurs in X-linked gammaglobulinaemia, common variable immunodeficiency, and IgA deficiency. Loss of T-cell function occurs in ataxia telangiectasia. Loss of both T-cell and antibody function leads to severe combined immunodeficiency. AIDS patients are prone to a wide variety of gastrointestinal infections (*Table 2*).

Pathophysiology
Normally, there is a highly specialized gut immune system consisting of:
- A surface layer of secretory IgA of the gut mucosa, specialized to resist digestion and providing protective immunity against gut flora.
- Cell-mediated immunity consisting of T-cells, between epithelial cells and in the lamina propria.
- Plasma cells (mainly IgA), producing IgA, which can be transported to the surface of the mucosa as secretory IgA.

Deficiencies may occur as a result of a genetic inability to produce IgA, acquired inability to make all classes of immunoglobulin (common variable hypogammaglobulinaemia), inability to make new immune responses (loss of helper T-cells in AIDS), destruction of immuno-competent cells (chemotherapy) or drug immunosuppression. Often, gastrointestinal manifestations of immunodeficiency coexist with generalized immunodeficiency (e.g. recurrent chest and sinus infections).

Clinical history
For immunoglobulin deficiency, check for a history of other systemic infections. Look also for risk factors for AIDS and/or a history of AIDS-related infections (e.g. oesophageal candidiasis).

Table 2 Main HIV-associated infections within the gastrointestinal tract

Mouth	• *Candida* • Hairy oral leukoplakia (Epstein–Barr(EBV)-related) • Herpes simplex virus (HSV) types 1 and 2 • Idiopathic ulceration
Oesophagus	• Candidal oesophagitis • EBV-related ulceration • CMV ulcers • HSV
Small bowel	• HIV enteropathy • *Mycobacterium avium intracellulare* complex • Giardiasis • *Cryptosporidium* • *Microsporidium* • *Isospora*
Liver	• *Mycobacterium avium intracellulare* complex and tuberculosis • Hepatitis B • Hepatitis C
Biliary tract	• Sclerosing cholangitis • CMV • *Cryptosporidium* • *Microsporidium*
Colon	• Colitis • CMV • *Campylobacter* • *Clostridium difficile* • *Salmonella* • *Mycobacterium avium intracellulare* complex and tuberculosis • *Blastocystis hominis*
Proctitis /perianal	• HSV • CMV • Warts
General	In addition, tumours (Kaposi's sarcoma, lymphoma) may occur in any site

Physical examination
In childhood, recurrent infections lead to poor development, weight loss, and malabsorption. Systemic immunodeficiencies may give rise to skin infections, and Kaposi's sarcoma in AIDS.

Special investigations

Check stool cultures and cultures of jejunal juice for infections. Carry out HIV antibody testing. Check serum immunoglobulins, lymphocyte count, T-cell count, jejunal biopsy, and staining for IgA, IgG, and IgM. Perform a small-bowel enema – in common variable hypogammaglobulinaemia there may be nodular lymphoid hyperplasia, reflecting abnormal aggregates of lymphatic cells (**154, 155**). Direct inspection of biopsies for infections (e.g. giardiasis, cryptosporidiosis, **156, 157**) should be made.

Prognosis

This is variable. In HIV infection, eradicating gut infection is difficult. In IgA deficiency, symptoms may be mild and transient. In severe cases of combined variable immunodeficiency – T-cell deficiencies in children – retarded growth and malnutrition may occur, reflecting malabsorption.

Management

Priorities include:
- Investigation of the underlying cause.
- Culture and biopsy to identify treatable organisms.

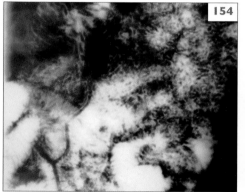

154 Small-intestinal follow-through, showing multiple nodular filling defects in the small intestine – nodular lymphoid hyperplasia – in common variable hypogammaglobulinaemia.

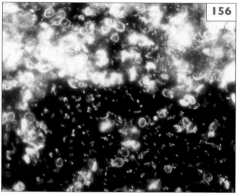

156 Dark-field view of upper intestinal contents in a patient with common variable hypergammaglobulinaemia – small 'tennis racket' outlines of *Giardia lamblia*.

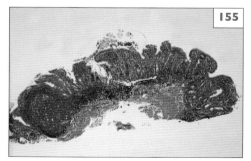

155 Small-intestinal biopsy in common variable hypogammaglobulinaemia and nodular lymphoid hyperplasia, showing prominent lymphoid follicle.

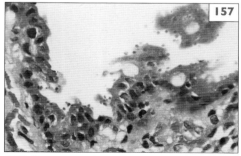

157 Cryptosporidia – round protozoa at the epithelial surface.

Lymphoma of the small intestine

Definition
This is a malignant disease of the lymphoid tissue of the small intestine.

Epidemiology and aetiology
Lymphoma of the small intestine is uncommon (as are tumours of the small intestine in general). There are a number of distinct types:
- Primary small-intestinal lymphoma with no pre-existing cause. The lymphoma is of B-cell origin, occurs generally in the ileum, in males more often than females, and in young adults or the elderly.
- Primary small-intestinal lymphoma with predisposing cause. These are of three subtypes:
  1. Lymphoma complicating adult coeliac disease – enteropathy-associated T-cell lymphoma in the upper small intestine.
  2. Lymphoma complicating chronic infection – 'Mediterranean lymphoma' of B-cells (IgA derived) in the upper small intestine (**158–162**). There is a strong geographic incidence (Middle East, Southern Africa, and in rural areas).
  3. Lymphoma complicating immunosuppression – seen in HIV infection or long-term immunosuppression.

- Secondary small-intestinal lymphoma – untreated or relapsing non-Hodgkin's lymphoma frequently affects the gut in its terminal stages.

Pathophysiology and aetiology
When a predisposing cause is identified, it appears that persistent antigenic challenge (gluten, multiple bacterial infection) leads to overexpression and development of a malignant clone of T- or B-cells. The pathophysiology reflects the nature of involvement, which may be diffuse (associated with wall thickening, loss of villous architecture, and obstruction of lymphatics) or may consist of single or multiple deposits in the gut wall, leading to local complications. The spread is from the gut to the mesenteric lymph nodes, more distant lymph nodes, and then systemically, including the liver and spleen.

Clinical history
When there is no previous gut involvement, presentations are most often surgical emergencies (obstruction, bleeding, or perforation). Diarrhoea, pain, and malabsorption are less common presentations. Relapse in coeliac disease, despite maintenance of a gluten-free diet, is a classical presentation.

Examination
This is variable. Findings may include a 'doughy' abdomen on palpation, and local masses. Hepatosplenomegaly and systemic lymphadenopathy are seen in advanced cases.

Laboratory and special examinations
Laboratory markers are often abnormal (high ESR, anaemia, hypoalbuminaemia) but nonspecific. IgA and IgA heavy chains should be sought (see below). Anatomical studies such as small-bowel enema may show irregular thickening of the wall, areas of narrowing or dilatation, and diffuse or localized ulceration. Ultrasound and CT may show evidence of wall thickening and define lymphadenopathy.

Histology is mandatory for diagnosis and may require laparotomy/laparoscopy and full-thickness biopsy to stage the disease.

Differential diagnosis
Crohn's disease and tuberculosis are the main differential diagnoses.

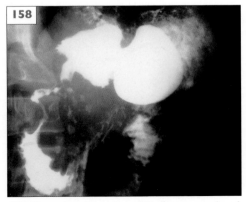

158 Extensive distortion of the first, second, and third part of the duodenum in a patient with upper intestinal lymphoma (Mediterranean type).

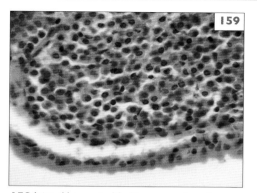

159 Jejunal biopsy in Mediterranean lymphoma showing infiltration with plasma cells (IgA-producing).

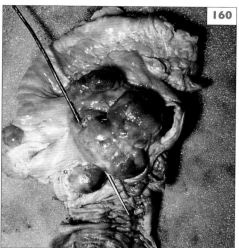

160 Nodular lymphoma (Mediterranean lymphoma) at autopsy.

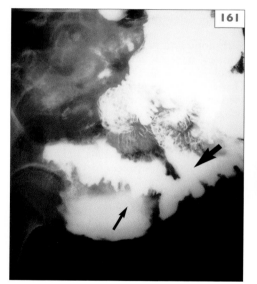

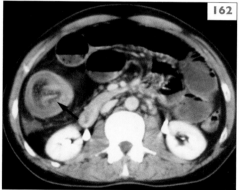

162 Gastrointestinal lymphoma presenting as the head of an intussusception (arrow).

161 Lymphoma of the distal terminal ileum showing irregular thickening (thick arrow) of the walls, and a shapeless abscess cavity (thin arrow) just below, as an indolent perforation has occurred.

Prognosis

Prognosis is generally poor, reflecting the late stage at which the diagnosis is usually made.

Management

Surgery is often essential, as the presentation may be with surgical emergency, requiring local resection of obviously diseased tissue. Surgery may be curative, but is rarely so due to diffuse gastrointestinal involvement and late presentation. Therefore, systemic chemotherapy is more generally used.

Special forms

The rare Mediterranean lymphoma involves proliferation of IgA-producing B-cells. Diagnosis may be helped by the identification of abnormal free IgA heavy chain (part of the Ig molecule) in serum or other fluids. At an early stage, this proliferation passes through an apparently benign form (immunoproliferative small-intestinal disease), in which antibiotic therapy (reducing the antigenic challenge in the gut) may lead to reversal of the condition.

Small-intestinal carcinoid tumours

Definition

These are tumours derived from enterochromaffin cells (a subtype of endocrine cell) of the small intestine.

Aetiology and epidemiology

Carcinoid tumours are very common, but clinical problems from them are rare, although possibly dramatic (**163**). Carcinoid tumours in the appendix (and rectum) are very common (up to 1% of the population), generally small and benign, and rarely symptomatic. Carcinoid tumours in the ileum, jejunum, or duodenum may also be benign, but are likely to become malignant. A number of those that are malignant secrete hormones and other substances, and give rise to the 'carcinoid syndrome'. Incidence is equal between sexes, and more common with advancing age, but can occur below the age of 30 years.

Pathology and pathophysiology

Primary tumours are smooth, submucosal nodules, which are generally asymptomatic. However, with growth they can ulcerate and bleed, or lead to subacute obstruction. If they become malignant, they infiltrate through the gut wall to the serosa, and spread to the lymph nodes and liver (**164**). In addition, they can be associated with local thickening and fibrosis of the gut wall and mesentery (desmoplasia) as a response to the tumour, making obstruction more likely (**165**). There are generally no systemic symptoms from release of hormones or other substances from primary tumours. If liver metastases occur, intermittent release into the circulation of substances such as serotonin can give rise to characteristics of carcinoid syndrome – flushing due to vasodilatation (**163**), and diarrhoea due to increased motility and gut secretion. In the long term, fibrosis of valves of the right side of the heart may lead to cardiac failure. In extreme cases, symptoms of pellagra may appear, due to diversion of B vitamins to synthesize serotonin.

Clinical history

With primary tumours, symptoms are as for other primary tumours – obstruction, bleeding, or incidentally found (e.g. at appendicectomy). With secondary tumours, presentation is either with hepatomegaly/pain (particularly with nonsecreting tumours) or with symptoms of carcinoid syndrome. Secondary carcinoid tumours may be very slow growing, so survival with secondaries may be 10–20 years (mean 3–5 years). In carcinoid syndrome, episodes of flushing and diarrhoea occur, with sweating and, in some patients, bronchoconstriction. With advanced disease, weight loss and cardiac failure may occur.

Physical examination

There is generally none at the primary stage. At the secondary stage, hepatomegaly (which may be huge), peripheral oedema, thickening of skin, facial flushing (**163**), conjunctivitis, permanent vasodilatation, and tricuspid and pulmonary stenosis should be looked for.

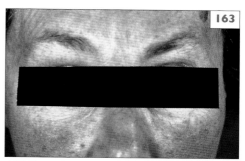

163 Face of a patient with carcinoid syndrome, showing flushing and telangiectasia.

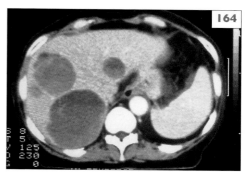

164 Large secondary deposits of carcinoid tumour in the liver on CT scan.

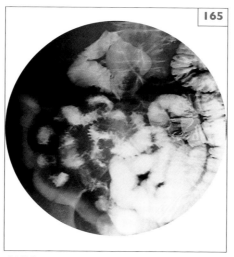

165 Extensive small-intestinal involvement with carcinoid primary in the terminal ileum. The distortion reflects fibrosis due to reaction in the tissues, not spread of the primary tumour itself.

Laboratory and special examinations

For primary tumours, small-bowel studies should be used. Indium 111-labelled octreotide scans are sometimes used in localizing the primary tumour (**166**).

For secondary tumours, ultrasound and CT should be used to identify deposits in the liver and mesentery. A biopsy should be taken to confirm diagnosis. For suspected carcinoid syndrome, the 24-hr urinary excretion of 5-hydroxyindoleacetic acid (5-HIAA, a metabolite of serotonin) should be monitored, together with serum gut hormones and serum chromogranin A (a protein coreleased from neuroendocrine tissue), which is also raised.

Differential diagnosis

* At the primary stage, differentiate from other small-intestinal tumours.
* At the secondary stage, differentiate from other metastatic disease in the liver.

Carcinoid tumours can arise in sites other than the small intestine, and have varying tendencies to become malignant (rectum generally benign, colon commonly malignant), although neither of these gives rise to carcinoid syndrome. Bronchial adenomas may give rise to carcinoid syndrome, and may also become malignant.

Prognosis

This is variable. Prognosis for appendiceal carcinoid is very good, and surgery is curative.

Management

For primary tumours without metastases, use a surgical approach.

In the case of carcinoid presenting with secondary deposits and no symptoms, management is difficult: chemotherapy or tumour debulking has not been demonstrated to prolong survival. For carcinoid syndrome, treatment depends on severity and consists of controlling hormonal effects (ciproheptadine, somatostatin, surgical debulking, or hepatic artery embolization to devascularize tumours) or of chemotherapy (interferon, streptozotocin, and 5-fluorouracil).

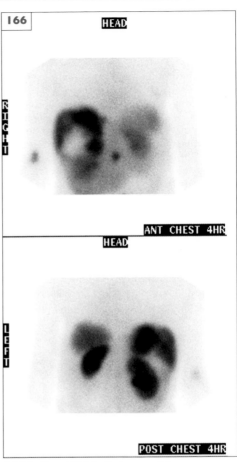

166 Indium 111-labelled octreotide scan showing uptake by carcinoid deposits.

Other intestinal tumours

BENIGN SMALL-INTESTINAL TUMOURS
Benign tumours of the small intestine are rare. They may be derived from smooth muscle cells (leiomyoma), fat cells (lipoma), or nerve elements (neuroma). They may present with obstruction or bleeding.

MALIGNANT SMALL-INTESTINAL TUMOURS
Primary malignant tumours of the small intestine are much rarer than in either the colon or stomach. The main types are:
- Cancers (**167, 168**).
- Carcinoid tumours (see above).
- Lymphomas (see above).

SMALL-INTESTINAL CANCERS
These occur occasionally with predisposing cause (Crohn's disease, coeliac disease). Other cases occur in patients who carry a familial genetic predisposition (family cancer syndromes) and have a strong family history of colonic, small-intestinal, breast, and ovarian cancer.

Pathophysiology
Local deposits of tumour spread and infiltrate from the epithelium through the gut wall, and metastasize to the lymph nodes and liver.

Clinical history
Presentation is with pain, obstruction, or bleeding. Small-intestinal tumours are so rare that there is generally considerable delay in making the diagnosis. Some patients present with unexplained anaemia.

Physical examination
This is only abnormal in advanced cases, with anaemia, local masses, subacute obstruction, and hepatomegaly.

Laboratory and special examinations
Anaemia may be present. A high ESR indicates probable local or distant spread. No 'specific' tumour markers occur in the serum. A small-intestinal radiograph is not always diagnostic, as tumours can be missed. Wireless capsule endoscopy is more sensitive. Angiography, particularly in investigating 'chronic gastrointestinal bleeding of unknown cause', may show vascular tumours. Laparotomy may be the final diagnostic test.

Prognosis
Prognosis is poor, due to late-stage presentation. The 5-year survival rate is less than 25%.

Treatment
Surgery is the main option. There is generally a poor response to adjuvant chemotherapy. Radiation is not helpful, as the doses required would damage the remaining gut.

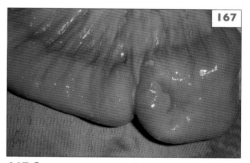

167 Operative specimen showing stenosis in the small intestine.

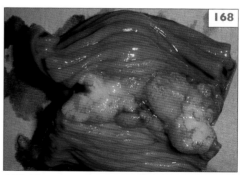

168 The same specimen as **167**. Here, in the opened specimen, the tumour causing the stenosis is now clearly seen.

Intestinal obstruction

Definition
The clinical picture is of obstruction of the intestinal lumen. This may be acute or subacute, and arise in the small or large intestine. It may be incomplete or complete.

Epidemiology and aetiology
There are multiple causes in childhood, including congenital stenosis, volvulus, and 'meconium ileus' in cystic fibrosis. In adults, the cause may be adhesions due to previous surgery. Tumours (**169**), hernias (**170**), and inflammatory processes (Crohn's disease of the small intestine, diverticular disease, and cancer of the colon) are other causes.

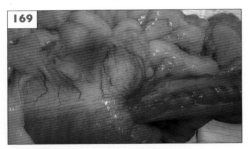

169 An uncommon cause of obstruction – operative specimen showing an intussuscepting cancer.

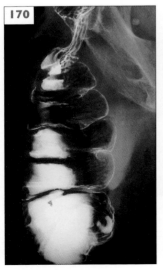

170 Hernias (particularly femoral hernias) should be remembered as causes of obstruction. This is a barium X-ray showing caecum prolapsing into a right inguinal hernia.

Pathophysiology
In intestinal obstruction, secretion of fluid is induced proximally, leading to a clinical picture of distension and fluid loss into the gut, and severe electrolyte disturbances.

Clinical history
The full-blown history of complete obstruction is colicky pain, distension, vomiting, and constipation. More proximal obstruction causes vomiting earlier; more distal obstruction causes absolute constipation earlier.

Physical examination
The patient should be examined for dehydration, abdominal distension, and visible peristalsis (**171**). A rectal examination (low carcinoma/faecal impaction in the elderly) is mandatory.

Investigations
General tests
These include electrolytes (increased urea and creatinine), hypokalaemia, and increased haemoglobin (representing dehydration). An initial blood screening should include crossmatching.

Specific tests
A plain abdominal radiograph is most revealing (**172**). A supine radiograph is essential, an erect radiograph helpful. The presentation of dilated loops (fluid levels on erect film) often permits definition of the site of obstruction. A gastrointestinal follow-through with conventional radiograph (or CT) can help to define the site of obstruction (**173–175**). In suspected low (colonic) obstruction, colonoscopy or barium enema may define the cause of obstruction from below, and barium enema should be performed before small-bowel radiography.

Management
Initial resuscitation and restoration of fluid balance (nasogastric tube, intravenous fluids) is vital, and allows time for further investigations. Unless symptoms resolve, surgery will be indicated, but definition of the cause is helpful. Pseudo-obstruction should be excluded.

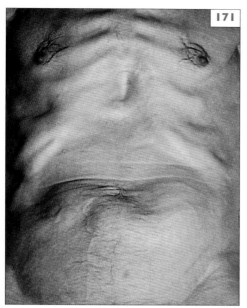

171 Small-intestinal obstruction – note the visible peristalsis.

172 Erect plain abdominal film of small-bowel obstruction.

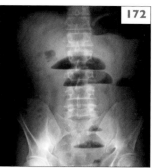

173 Duodenal obstruction – it is difficult to see where the stomach ends and the duodenum begins, but there is clearly obstruction in the duodenum.

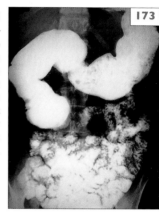

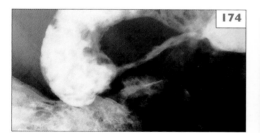

174 The obstruction in 173 is due to a narrow segment of Crohn's disease in the third part of duodenum, shown in this film.

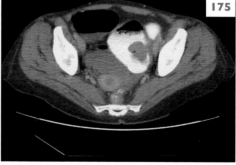

175 CT showing tumour arising at the site of bowel anastomosis in Crohn's disease.

Pseudo-obstruction

Definition

The clinical picture is suggestive of obstruction in the absence of an obstruction to the gut lumen (**176**). One particular form is 'paralytic ileus', which involves distended fluid-filled, nonmobile loops of gut, most often seen after prolonged manipulation of the gut during surgery. Paralysis may also occur as a result of neglected small-bowel obstruction.

Aetiology

Cases typically occur in:
- Elderly, debilitated patients with severe illness (sepsis, circulatory failure).
- Patients with chronic disease affecting neural or neuromuscular supply of the gut (familial visceral neuropathy, familial visceral myopathy).
- Patients with retroperitoneal tumour.

The symptoms reflect a combination of loss of motility and secondary bacterial overgrowth.

Clinical history

In severe illness, vomiting and distension may occur, and differential diagnosis is that of organic bowel obstruction. In chronic pseudo-obstruction, patients present with distension, occasionally vomiting, and intermittent pain, and may have either constipation or diarrhoea.

Investigations

The initial investigation is definition of patency of the entire gastrointestinal tract by contrast radiology, usually also showing slow transit. Biopsies may show abnormal muscle or absent nerves, but are often problematic. A full-thickness biopsy may be required. Conventional histology may be normal.

Prognosis

Acute pseudo-obstruction following surgery will usually resolve with careful fluid balance and withdrawal of drugs such as opiates, which slow gut motility. In more prolonged cases, colonoscopic decompression has been advocated, as has neostigmine. Progressive familial forms lead to malnutrition and may eventually require total parenteral nutrition. Repeated surgery is a hazard. Little can be done surgically, because postoperative ileus makes things worse. Episodes are worse with bacterial overgrowth, and intermittent antibiotic treatment may help.

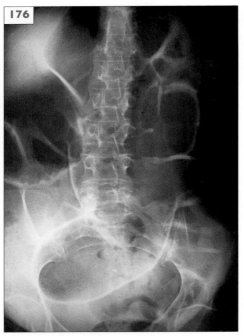

176

176 Gross dilatation of the large and small bowel. This patient has a chronic pseudo-obstruction caused by a visceral myopathy.

Infections of the small intestine

VIRAL GASTROENTERITIS

This is an acute condition with nausea, vomiting, and diarrhoea, generally self-limited (1–3 days). It is usually suspected rather than formally diagnosed. Causes are rotavirus, calicivirus, astrovirus, and Norwalk agent. The condition should be treated symptomatically. If diarrhoea is present, oral replacement of fluids and electrolytes can prevent dehydration without the use of intravenous fluids.

PROTOZOAL INFECTIONS

Giardiasis

Giardia lamblia (**137**) is a protozoal pathogen, transmitted by oral/faecal contamination. It contaminates the upper small intestine, and presents acutely with nausea, diarrhoea, and weight loss. This may initiate a chronic malabsorptive state, particularly in immunodeficiency. Diagnosis is by analysis of duodenal fluid, duodenal biopsy, or (least efficient) cysts in the stool. Generally, responses to treatment with metronidazole are adequate, but repeat treatment may be necessary.

Cryptosporidiosis

Cryptosporidium (**138**) is a waterborne protozoon, which can cause acute self-limited diarrhoea in otherwise healthy people. The main clinical relevance is in the immunocompromised (notably AIDS patients), where it can cause protracted diarrhoea. It is identified histologically on light microscopy. Treatment with spiramycin is generally unsatisfactory.

BACTERIAL INFECTIONS

Salmonellosis

A wide variety of species of *Salmonella* give rise to acute enteritis. Systemic infections occur (with invasion) with *S. typhi* and *S. paratyphi*, resulting in generalized fever and abdominal pain, often with constipation in the early stages and diarrhoea in the late stages (second week). Invasion is via the terminal ileum lymphoid tissue. Perforation may occur.

Diagnosis

Diagnosis is by culture of blood, faeces, and urine. Serology (Widal test) is generally unreliable.

Treatment

Treatment is with ampicillin, ciprofloxacin, or chloramphenicol. Noninvasive *Salmonella* (e.g. *S. typhimurium*) gives enteritis with fever and diarrhoea, only occasionally with bleeding. Paradoxically, antibiotics may lead to prolongation of carriage. Diagnosis is performed on stool culture.

Campylobacter enteritides

Campylobacter (see Chapter 8) is a common cause of acute diarrhoea, with both small-intestinal and colonic colonization. Presentation is with bloody diarrhoea, and marked intestinal cramps and fever, often in small epidemics. Outbreaks frequently arise from the ingestion of poorly cooked chicken. The condition is rarely invasive and is generally self-limited. It should be treated with antibiotics only if severe.

Cholera

Vibrio cholerae is a bacterial, waterborne infection, which is the cause of potentially devastating epidemics, particularly in the Third World and after civil or military upheaval. *Vibrio cholerae* toxin binds to the surface of the enterocyte and induces secretion of sodium-rich fluid into the small intestine, mainly by activation of cyclic AMP. The gut mucosa is not significantly inflamed. The result is many litres of fluid loss and diarrhoea, characteristically seen as the cholereic 'rice-water' stool.

Treatment

Correction of fluid balance is the primary aim. Despite major activation of enterocyte secretion, the absorption capacity of cells is intact, so rather than intravenous therapy (which is often impracticable in cholera conditions), the use of 'cholera-replacement fluids' or oral rehydration fluids is recommended. These activate the glucose-dependent sodium pump. The typical constitution is: sodium, 90 mmol/l; glucose, 111 mmol/l; potassium, 20 mmol/l; and citrate, 10 mmol/l. Antibiotics (tetracycline, trimethoprim-sulphamethoxazole) are also indicated, but there is increasing resistance to these.

Oral rehydration fluids have been used extensively for treatment of all kinds of infectious diarrhoea (not only cholera), particularly in the Third World, and represent a triumph of applied physiology.

TUBERCULOSIS ENTERITIS

This is a chronic infection caused by *Mycobacterium tuberculosis*. Both human and bovine strains can cause the disease. An atypical *Mycobacterium* can cause infection, particularly in the immunosuppressed. In the absence of immunosuppression, cases of tuberculous enteritis are rare in the West, except in immigrants. The condition is common in the developing world and may occur with or without pulmonary involvement. It occurs most often in the ileocaecal region (**177**, **178**) (differential diagnosis is Crohn's disease), but can also occur as diffuse upper small-intestinal disease (multiple strictures) or colonic disease.

Clinical manifestations

The condition presents with pain, diarrhoea, obstruction, or colonic bleeding, with variable weight loss. Ascites may be present (tuberculous peritonitis). Pulmonary tuberculosis is not always present.

Diagnosis and management

Contrast radiology shows an abnormal inflamed, irregular wall of the gut and strictures. A biopsy should be taken endoscopically if possible. Merely finding the *Mycobacterium* in the stool is misleading (environmental mycobacteria may also be found), so specific identification is necessary. On suspicion, treatment is with conventional antituberculous drugs.

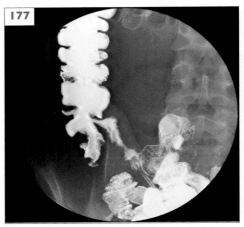

177 Tuberculosis – barium study showing contraction and distortion of the caecum.

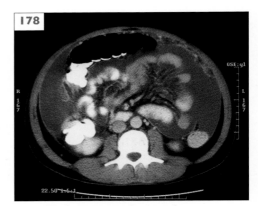

178 CT of a patient with ascites from tuberculosis involving gut and peritoneum.

CESTODES (TAPEWORMS)
Segmented flatworms
These include:
- *Taenia saginata* – beef tapeworm.
- *Taenia solium* – pork tapeworm.
- *Hymenolepsis nana* – dwarf tapeworm.
- *Diphyllobothrium latum* – fish tapeworm.

Human ingestion of infected meat or fish containing larval forms results in infestation of the small intestine. The worms stays anchored to the wall of the intestine by suckers or spikes sited on its head (or scolex). The worms are segmented and eggs develop in the segments: stool examination may reveal intact segments (proglottides) and eggs. The existence of adult worms is often asymptomatic, although obstruction may occur rarely. Pig tapeworm larvae may invade in humans, leading to cysticercosis, which affects the CNS and muscles. Niclosamide is the best treatment for intestinal infestation. Praziquantel treats both intestinal and systemic larval infestation.

Strongyloidiasis
Strongyloides worms colonize the upper gastrointestinal tract (**179, 180**). In the immunosuppressed, or if there are anatomical abnormalities such as diverticulae, the worm can complete its whole reproductive cycle in the human tract. Hyperinfestation can lead to obstruction and bacterial septicaemia, with worms carrying bacteria into the body as they invade the mucosa. The infection commences by larvae penetrating the skin, trafficking to the lungs (causing pulmonary infiltration), and thence passing via the trachea to the oesophagus down to the duodenum where the adult worms develop. They may cause pain, diarrhoea, malabsorption, and eosinophilia. Treatment is with thiabendazole, but eradication is difficult if there is anatomical abnormality or immunosuppression.

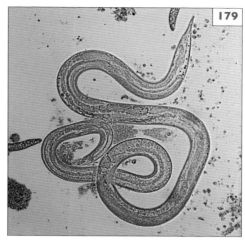

179 *Strongyloides stercoralis* – a worm colonizing the upper small intestine.

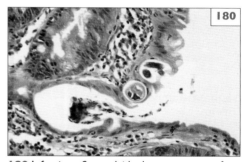

180 Infectious *Strongyloides* larvae, a cause of malabsorption in the immunosuppressed.

Vascular disease of the small intestine

Definition
A number of types of primary vascular pathology cause small-intestinal disease.

Arteriosclerotic disease
This rarely causes gastrointestinal disturbance, unless two of the three major arteries to the gut (coeliac, superior mesenteric, and inferior mesenteric artery) are completely or partially occluded (**181, 182**). Normally, the rich collateral supply protects the small intestine, which is less susceptible to damage than the colon. Possible symptoms are:
- Mesenteric angina – pain after eating, leading to weight loss.
- Acute infarction (**183**) – precipitated by embolization (atrial fibrillation, artificial valves, mural thrombosis after myocardial infarct) – causes pain and paralytic ileus, and may lead to intestinal perforation or localized peritonitis. In addition, low-flow states (e.g. heart failure) can cause paralytic ileus.

Venous thrombosis
This may occur:
- In low-flow states.
- In hypercoagulable states, e.g. polycythaemia, deficiency of endogenous anticoagulants (protein C, protein S, antithrombin III, factor V Leiden).
- Secondary to severe dehydration.

The condition leads to pain and gastrointestinal bleeding as a result of venous congestion. This may lead to portal venous obstruction, and the development of portal systemic collaterals, including oesophageal varices.

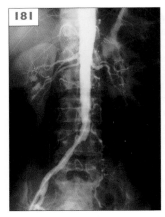

181 Anterior arteriogram showing renal arteries, but absence of left iliac, inferior mesenteric, and superior mesenteric arteries.

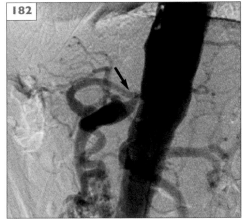

182 Aortogram in a patient with mesenteric angina. There is stenosis of the origin of the coeliac axis on the anterior side of the aorta (arrow).

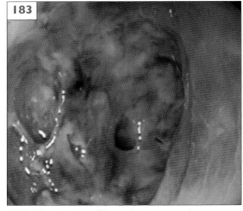

183 Necrotic small bowel seen at endoscopy.

VASCULITIDES

Collagen vascular disorders can affect small and medium-sized arteries of the small intestine (polyarteritis nodosa, **184**; Behçet's disease; lupus erythematosus), causing pain and bleeding, but rarely perforation and late complication of a stricture. The colon can also be involved (with a scenario as for colitis). The most common vasculitis is Henoch–Schönlein purpura – a response to exogenous antigens (e.g. *Streptococcus*, some foods). This gives a triad of:

* Skin rash (**185**).
* Acute glomerulonephritis (red cell casts in urine, increase in blood pressure, oedema).
* Gastrointestinal involvement – terminal ileum inflammation with pain (often due to intussusception) and bleeding (**186**).

Most cases of Henoch–Schönlein purpura resolve spontaneously, although on occasion corticosteroids may be indicated. A minority of patients progresses to renal failure.

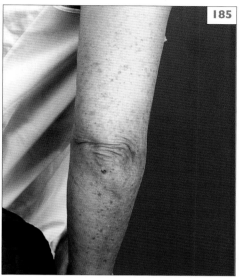

185 Vasculitis area on the extensor surfaces in Henoch–Schönlein purpura.

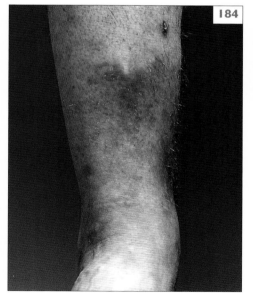

184 Systemic vasculitis with nodular involvement of the skin.

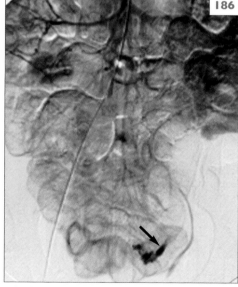

186 Superior mesenteric angiogram showing a bleed in the ileum secondary to vasculitis.

Pancreas

Symptomatically it may be difficult to recognize that the pancreas is abnormal

Acute pancreatitis is a major medical emergency

Chronic pancreatitis may be difficult to diagnose

Pancreatic cancer often presents late, yet early diagnosis is vital if there is to be a chance of cure

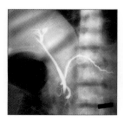 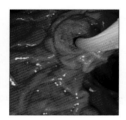 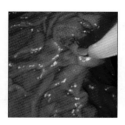 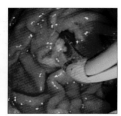

Anatomy and histology

The pancreas lies transversely across the abdomen retroperitoneally. Its ductal system reflects its embryonic origin and occasionally there may be two openings of pancreatic ducts into the duodenum (the ampulla of Vater and accessory ampulla). The pancreatic head, body, and tail drain through the pancreatic duct into the duodenum.

Histology

The pancreatic acini, which secrete pancreatic enzymes, drain into the pancreatic ductules and then the duct. The islets of Langerhans are 'neuroendocrine tissues', which are scattered throughout the pancreatic parenchyma.

Investigations

These include imaging of pancreatic morphology and functional tests.

Imaging
Plain radiograph
This is frequently normal, but in chronic pancreatitis it may show pancreatic calcification. In the assessment of a patient with acute pancreatitis, an isolated ileus of the small intestine ('sentinel loop') can occasionally be seen.

Barium radiograph
This is of little use, unless pancreatic inflammation or tumour distorts the second and third parts of the duodenum.

Ultrasound, CT scans
These may show enlargement or irregularity of the pancreas, surrounding inflammation, and the presence of cysts, pseudocysts, mass lesions, or dilatation of ducts. Transabdominal ultrasound may be difficult, due to overlying gas.

Endoscopic ultrasound
EUS affords excellent pancreatic visualization, and the opportunity to biopsy lesions.

Magnetic resonance cholangiopancreatography
MRCP has become the primary means to image the pancreatic and larger bile ducts. Images acquired in this way are now a key noninvasive anatomical investigation. MRCP has superseded the use of ERCP as the preferred technique to image the pancreatic ducts. Examples of MRCP are shown in Chapter 7.

Tissue sampling
Endoscopic retrograde cholangiopancreatography
ERCP (**187, 188**) maintains its value for tissue sampling and endoscopic intervention (predominantly in the biliary tract). A side-viewing endoscope is orientated towards the ampulla, and cannulated – selecting either the bile duct or pancreatic duct. Radio-opaque contrast is introduced into the ducts, and used to identify the ducts and abnormalities. Biopsy samples and cytology specimens (brushings) are taken as appropriate. Therapeutic procedures, such as extraction of bile duct stones and insertion of stents, are undertaken. ERCP is the key interventional investigation in pancreatico-biliary disease; with respect to the pancreas, it should show the normal duct, duct distortion, or dilatation in chronic pancreatitis, obstruction, or tumour mass.

Direct percutaneous fine needle aspiration and/or biopsy of pancreatic masses
This can be performed under ultrasound (endoscopic or transabdominal) or CT guidance.

Endoscopic ultrasound
EUS is increasingly used in staging pancreatic tumours and selecting patients for surgery. EUS-guided fine needle aspiration or core biopsy

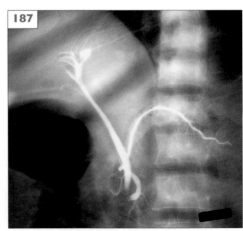

187 Normal pancreatic duct and biliary duct shown at ERCP.

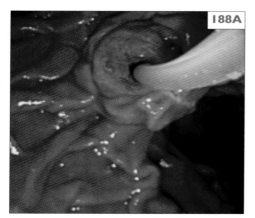

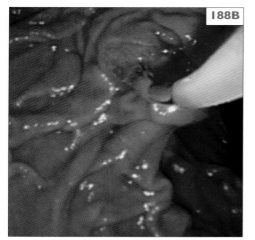

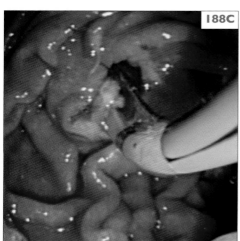

of suspicious lesions can also be undertaken. It is safer than percutaneous biopsy, and has the theoretical advantage that the biopsy track passes through the tissue eventually excised at surgery. This reduces the opportunity for tumour seeding. EUS is very sensitive to the early changes of chronic pancreatitis.

Functional tests

These rely on evidence of pancreatic exocrine function and are now rarely performed.

Tube tests

These include the Lundh test meal and secretin test. They require duodenal intubation and recovery of pancreatic juice after a test meal, or injection of the hormone secretin to stimulate pancreatic secretion. Classical results in chronic pancreatitis show a normal volume of dilute pancreatic juice, i.e. low bicarbonate secretion and low protein. In cancer of the pancreas, results show a small volume of normal pancreatic juice (although these groups often overlap). These tests are now rarely used.

Tubeless tests

Here, a substrate given by mouth is broken down by active pancreatic enzymes. For example, the para-aminobenzoic acid (PABA) test uses PABA bound to fluorescein, given by mouth. If digested normally, the fluorescein is split off and secreted in the urine. Excretion >30% is taken as normal.

Detection of pancreatic enzymes in stool

This is another means to investigate exocrine pancreatic function. Measurement of faecal elastase correlates well with invasive tests of pancreatic exocrine function, and is convenient for patients. Unlike the PABA or pancreolauryl tests, it does not require 24-hr urine collections.

188 ERCP sequence showing: (**A**) access to bile duct and (**B, C**) the sphincterotomy.

Acute pancreatitis

Definition
This is a clinical syndrome characterized by acute inflammation of the pancreas. Abdominal pain and abnormal serum pancreatic enzyme levels are typical.

Epidemiology and aetiology
All populations are affected, although with significant variability related to the prevalence of predisposing causes. Cholelithiasis (including microlithiasis) and, particularly, bile duct stones, constitute the single largest cause (30–85% of cases), increasing the risk by 12- to 35-fold. Alcohol is implicated in approximately 5% of cases of acute pancreatitis. In chronic alcoholics, acute-on-chronic pancreatitis is a common problem. Other causes include trauma, drugs (e.g. azathioprine, pentamidine, or thiazide diuretics), infectious agents (e.g. mumps, HIV), hyperlipidaemia (triglycerides, usually >500 mg/dl, and hypercalcaemia. ERCP can precipitate pancreatitis, but rarely (0.4–1.2% of cases).

Pathophysiology
The precise mechanisms are complex. Pancreatic ductal obstruction is involved. Trypsinogen activation within the pancreatic acinar cells, impaired secretion of enzymes, and cell autodigestion all occur. These lead to interstitial oedema, inflammatory cell infiltration, tissue necrosis, and may lead on to damage to contiguous or distant organs and multiorgan failure.

Clinical history
Abdominal pain is most frequent, usually in the epigastric or umbilical region, with radiation to the back. Classically, pain is relieved by sitting and leaning forward, although this is uncommon. The pain may be extremely severe, may not peak for several hours, and is usually not relieved by vomiting. Nausea and vomiting are generally present. In advanced or severe pancreatitis, confusion, coma, or respiratory failure may occur.

Physical examination
Typical findings are tachycardia, hypotension, and fever. High-grade fever may be encountered with cholangitis or severe tissue necrosis. Jaundice is usually absent. Severe jaundice may indicate biliary obstruction or liver disease. Shock may be present. Abdominal tenderness, rigidity, and sluggish or absent bowel sounds may be found. Retroperitoneal haemorrhage may discolour the skin around the umbilicus (Cullen's sign) or flanks (Grey Turner's sign). Rarely, subcutaneous fat necrosis by circulating pancreatic enzymes may manifest with painful nodules (panniculitis).

Laboratory and special examinations
Biochemical tests
There is increased serum amylase level (specificity approximately 95% when serum amylase is more than three-fold that of normal subjects). Serum lipase (more specific) is the best enzyme marker. Serum amylase and lipase levels rise simultaneously early; serum amylase may return to normal within 24 hr, whereas serum lipase remains elevated for several days. Enzyme isoforms, such as L2 pancreatic lipase or pancreatic amylase, enhance specificity. The renal clearance of amylase may be increased by tubular dysfunction and is not diagnostic. Acute phase reactants, such as neutrophil elastase, interleukin-6, or CRP, are nonspecific. Serum bilirubin, aspartate aminotransferase (AST), alanine aminotransferase (ALT), and alkaline phosphatase help evaluate coexisting biliary disease.

Radiology
- Plain radiographs of the chest and abdomen should be used for detecting pleural effusion, 'sentinel loop' (**189**), or a perforation.
- Abdominal ultrasound should be used for gallstones or gallbladder 'sludge', although intestinal gas or obesity often limits pancreatic imaging.
- CT is often necessary, and demonstrates necrosis and/or extrapancreatic fluid collection (**190**). MRI has greater sensitivity than CT for detecting milder disease, and is superior for differentiating fluid collections, necrosis, and haemorrhage.
- MRI will delineate ductal anatomy, but ERCP is indicated in the acute setting for ductal trauma or obstruction, e.g. by gallstones and parasites. EUS will detect stones in the bile ducts, and is very sensitive for detecting biliary microlithiasis.

Differential diagnosis
Other causes of acute abdomen
These include acute cholecystitis, perforated peptic ulcer, acute intestinal obstruction, nephrolithiasis, ruptured aneurysm of abdominal

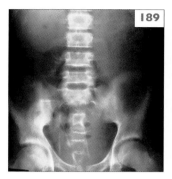

189 Acute pancreatitis – note the sentinel loop of jejunum next to the pancreas.

190 CT of acute pancreatitis – note swollen and necrotic pancreas (there is also ascites).

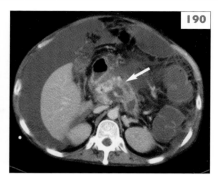

aorta, ruptured liver abscess or tumour, acute salpingo-oophoritis, etc.

Disease of other organs
These include lobar pneumonia, pleural disease, and CNS disease, e.g. subarachnoid haemorrhage when confusion or coma is predominant.

Abnormal serum amylase
In addition to acute pancreatitis, this indicates renal disease, salivary gland disease, and other acute abdominal events (including perforation of a duodenal ulcer). Salivary amylase rises in diabetic ketoacidosis. Macroamylasaemia in association with another cause for abdominal pain may be particularly confusing. In macroamylasaemia, large complexes of amylase and immunoglobulins, or amylase polymers, cannot be cleared by renal tubules and circulate in the blood. The diagnosis is established by demonstrating low renal amylase clearance, and by gel filtration to demonstrate macroamylase.

Prognosis
The prognosis is highly variable, ranging from uneventful recovery to multiple complications, protracted course and death.

The Ranson or Glasgow criteria utilize age, white blood cell count (WBC), lactate dehydrogenase (LDH), glucose, AST, albumin, calcium, arterial pO_2, and blood urea, at admission and within 48 hr to assign prognosis.

The Acute Physiology and Chronic Health Evaluation (APACHE) III criteria use 14 routinely measured parameters, and can be more quickly obtained.

The CT Severity Index is based upon pancreatic enlargement, extent of inflammation, peripancreatic fluid collection, and degree of tissue necrosis, and correlates with observations at surgery, as well as with the Ranson criteria.

In 80% of cases, patients have mild acute pancreatitis and improve within 48–72 hr. A minority runs a severe course, with attendant local complications and risk of multiorgan failure.

Early complications include fluid and electrolyte imbalances, gastrointestinal haemorrhage, shock, adult respiratory distress syndrome, and renal failure. Late complications include pancreatic ascites, pancreatic abscess, pseudocyst, or fistula (see 'Complications of pancreatitis').

Management
The mainstays are supportive care, treatment of the underlying cause, and prevention of complications. No curative treatments are available. Replacement of fluid and electrolyte deficits, and correction of metabolic abnormalities are important. Nasogastric aspiration is of unproven value, except when ileus exists. Protein intake is generally restricted and proteins are gradually reintroduced. Enteral feeding via a naso-jejunal feeding tube is usual; a period of intravenous hyperalimentation may be required if this not tolerated. Antibiotics may be necessary for complications. In gallstone pancreatitis, endoscopic papillotomy is indicated in those with jaundice or biliary sepsis. Emergency pancreatic surgery or inhibitors of pancreatic secretion are not generally indicated, although in severe disease with complications, such as abscesses or extensive pancreatic necrosis, surgery may be required.

Chronic pancreatitis

Definition
This is progressive and permanent pancreatic damage, resulting in tissue loss, morphological change, and/or abnormal function. Several classifications have been proposed based upon aetiology, clinical presentation, and morphological change, such as pancreatic fibrosis, obstruction, and calcification.

Epidemiology and aetiology
Prevalence is ill-defined, and varies widely among populations. One Western survey of the annual incidence of chronic pancreatitis was 8 per 100,000, with a prevalence of 26 per 100,000. Prolonged alcohol intake is the most frequent cause (approximately 70%). Idiopathic pancreatitis (10–40%) may present in younger (second-decade) or older (sixth-decade) age groups. Other causes (<10%) include tropical pancreatitis, hereditary pancreatitis, hyperparathyroidism, mechanical obstruction of the main pancreatic duct, and trauma.

Pathophysiology
The characteristic features are inflammatory changes, progressive atrophy (starting in acinar tissue and followed by the pancreatic islets), and fibrosis. The pancreatic ducts are dilated, particularly in the 'obstructive' form. The 'lithogenic' type is marked by intraductal plugs or stones and chronic calcification of the pancreas (**191, 192**). There is altered secretion of pancreatic enzymes, which promotes the autodigestion of tissues. Increased viscosity of pancreatic juice aids plug formation, ductal obstruction, and fibrosis. Pain is probably related to intrapancreatic distension and release of local neurotransmitters.

Clinical history
Abdominal pain is most common. The pain is epigastric, dull, and constant, radiates to the back, is worsened by food, and occurs in bouts lasting several days or weeks interspersed with pain-free intervals. Pain may continue unchanged, disappear, or decrease with the onset of pancreatic calcification or steatorrhoea. The latter occurs when enzyme secretion is reduced by >90%, usually after 10–20 years. Diabetes mellitus may develop between 5 and 18 years after the onset of pancreatitis. In 15% of cases, chronic pancreatitis may be painless. Other symptoms include nausea, vomiting, anorexia, weight loss due to fear of pain upon eating, malabsorption, jaundice, ascites, and pleural effusion.

Physical examination
Patients should be examined for cachexia (evidence of weight loss), epigastric tenderness, and occasionally abdominal distension in the setting of complications, such as pseudocyst.

Laboratory and special examinations
Serum amylase levels are usually normal. In severe disease, there may be a lower rise in serum pancreatic polypeptide levels in response to a protein test-meal or intravenous secretin. Tests of exocrine pancreatic function are of limited value. This is because duodenal intubation is necessary for sampling pancreatic juice, results may vary from laboratory to laboratory, and unequivocal abnormalities require extensive disease.

Tubeless tests of pancreatic insufficiency can be used, depending on local availability. Faecal elastase testing is also useful.

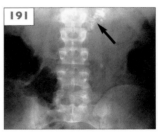

191 Plain abdominal X-ray showing calcification in the pancreas (arrow) (chronic pancreatitis).

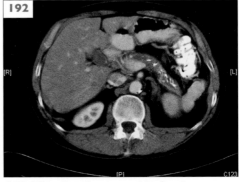

192 CT in chronic pancreatitis, showing calcification in the pancreatic body.

Pancreatic imaging

In 30–40% of patients, a plain radiograph or other X-ray imaging will show diffuse, speckled calcification (**191, 192**). In this case, no further testing is necessary. Ultrasound and CT (sensitivity and specificity approximately 90%) may show a small pancreas with altered texture, dilated main pancreatic duct (>4 mm), oedema, cavities, calcification, and pseudocysts.

Pancreatic ductal changes at ERCP may be graded into minimal (minor duct dilatation, intraductal calculi), moderate (dilated, tortuous, or stenotic main pancreatic duct), or advanced (addition of cystic changes) pancreatitis (**193–196**). However, normal findings at ERCP do not exclude chronic pancreatitis.

Endoscopic ultrasound

Changes in the pancreatic parenchyma and ductal system are readily detectable with EUS, and scoring systems have been developed. EUS is more sensitive than other imaging for the earliest changes of chronic pancreatitis, and does not have the morbidity of ERCP. It is valuable in differentiating focal chronic pancreatitis from pancreatic carcinoma.

Differential diagnosis

Differentiate from pancreatic carcinoma, intraductal papillary mucinous tumours, acid peptic disease, biliary disease, and occult malignancy.

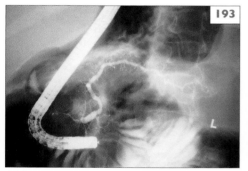

193 Minor irregularities of the ducts in a patient with chronic pancreatitis.

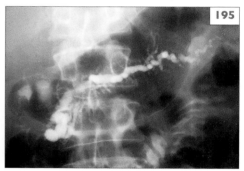

195 Severe chronic pancreatitis seen after ERCP (endoscope removed); there is a widened ectatic, tortuous pancreatic duct.

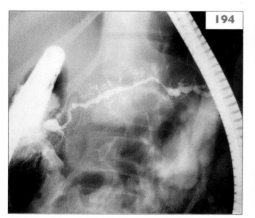

194 ERCP in a patient with chronic pancreatitis with 'string of lakes' appearance of pancreatic duct.

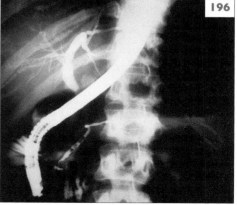

196 ERCP showing the pancreatic duct and the presence of intraductal calculi. The biliary tract is also demonstrated.

Prognosis

Chronic pancreatitis is an indolent disorder with periodic symptomatic exacerbations, leading over a number of years to total organ failure. There is a greater risk of pancreatic carcinoma. Obstructive biliary complications or other complications (see below) increase morbidity. Chronic alcoholism also predisposes to other diseases, such as infectious complications. Addiction to narcotic analgesics may pose difficulties.

Management

The mainstays are pain relief and improved nutritional status. Dietitians will advise patients to take small, frequent low-fat meals, sometimes with supplements of medium-chain fatty acids, which are directly absorbed. Specific deficiencies of fat-soluble vitamins may occur in patients with gross steatorrhoea. Abstinence from alcohol is helpful in the long term, but does not reverse the disease.

Pain management can be problematic; non-narcotic analgesics are used where possible, although opiates are usually necessary.

Oral replacement of pancreatic enzymes reduces steatorrhoea and diminishes pancreatic stimulation, intraductal pressure, pain, and malabsorption. Simultaneous gastric acid suppression and use of enteric-coated formulations improves the efficacy of enzyme replacement. EUS-guided injection of alcohol – and/or local anaesthetic – into the coeliac ganglion may help refractory pain, although the benefit lasts for only 3–6 months.

Endoscopic therapy

This is appropriate for papillary stenosis, stricture, or stone. The approaches include sphincterotomy, pancreatic-duct stenting, or balloon dilatation.

Surgery

Usually, the pancreas is diffusely involved in chronic pancreatitis. Surgery may benefit the minority of patients with localized ductal obstruction. Partial pancreatic resection is occasionally performed, as is pancreatico-jejunostomy.

Inherited pancreatic disorders

CYSTIC FIBROSIS

Cystic fibrosis (CF) is the commonest inherited pancreatic disorder, and is characterized by abnormally viscid exocrine secretions due to defective activation of a cAMP-dependent chloride channel.

Epidemiology and aetiology

An autosomal recessive disorder, CF is transmitted in 1 per 2,500 live Caucasian births. The gene frequency approaches 5% in northern Europeans. CF is also prevalent in southern Europeans, Ashkenazi Jews, and African Americans. Heterozygote carriers are asymptomatic. Abnormality of the CF gene affects the cystic fibrosis transmembrane conductance regulator (CFTR) – a number of mutations have been described. Normally, the cAMP-dependent CFTR in apical cell membranes of epithelial or duct cells allows the flow of chloride and bicarbonate, which leads to net fluid secretion and alkalinization. In CF, there is defective dilution and alkalinization of exocrine secretions, including those in pancreatic ducts, bile ducts, bronchial epithelium, and sweat glands.

Pathophysiology

There is increased viscosity of exocrine secretions and increased electrolyte concentrations in sweat and saliva. The consequences include intrauterine growth retardation, impaired foetal development, meconium ileus (obstruction of the neonatal gut), recurrent respiratory infection, bronchiectasis, chronic obstructive pulmonary disease, focal biliary cirrhosis, pancreatic exocrine insufficiency, and male genital tract lesions in the ductal systems. The pancreas is small, irregular, and cystic with eosinophilic duct concretions. Dilatation of ducts, enzyme leaks, and cycles of autodigestion lead to fat, fibrosis, and cystic changes, eventually impairing pancreatic islet function. Pancreatic insufficiency develops in >80% of patients, with gallbladder disease in 50% and gallstones in 12%.

Clinical history

Diarrhoea and steatorrhoea are the most common gastroenterological findings.

Physical examination

No specific abdominal abnormalities may be detected. Cholestasis may be associated with mild to moderate hepatomegaly. Biliary cirrhosis may develop.

Laboratory and special examinations

The diagnosis is made clinically by increased sweat Na^+ and Cl^- concentrations (>77 mmol/l and >74 mmol/l, respectively) and confirmed by molecular genetic methods. Steatorrhoea may be demonstrated by analysis of stool fat. Imaging modalities of ultrasound, CT and ERCP are employed as discussed at the beginning of the chapter.

Differential diagnosis

Differentiate from other causes of pancreatic insufficiency (particularly Schwachman's syndrome).

Prognosis

With improving attention to respiratory complications, median survival has increased to 29 years. Some patients survive to the fifth decade. The most critical factor is to prevent dehydration and infectious respiratory events.

Management

Pancreatic insufficiency is managed in the standard fashion. The goals are to relieve pain and steatorrhoea. Efforts towards effective gene therapy are aimed at expressing normal copies of the *CFTR* gene in affected epithelia.

SHWACHMAN'S SYNDROME

This is the second most common pancreatic disorder in children. It is an autosomal recessive condition, caused by mutation in the Shwachman–Bodian–Diamond syndrome (*SBDS*) gene, affecting 1 in 20,000 births. In addition to pancreatic exocrine insufficiency, abnormalities include haematological findings (cyclical neutropenia, anaemia, thrombocytopenia, or pancytopenia), bone disorders (metaphyseal dysostosis, short stature), eczema, diabetes mellitus, and Hirschsprung's disease. Failure to thrive and steatorrhoea occur. The pancreas is small and fatty. Infection is an important cause of mortality. Treatment is mainly supportive. Symptoms may spontaneously improve with age in some patients.

HEREDITARY PANCREATITIS

This is a familial syndrome, characterized by recurrent pancreatitis from early childhood and throughout life. The disorder is autosomal dominant, with a high penetrance (approximately 80%), and accounts for 5–10% of chronic pancreatitis cases. In some patients, deficiency of a pancreatic lithoprotein (which normally inhibits pancreatic stone formation) is believed to be involved; in other cases, there are mutations in the cationic trypsinogen gene. The mean age of onset is 10 years. The clinical presentation is characterized by prolonged attacks of pain, large calculi in major pancreatic ducts, frequent pancreatic calcification, and an increased incidence of pancreatic adenocarcinoma – some authorities suggest screening (CT and EUS) from the age of 35 years.

Complications of pancreatitis

The onset may be acute or insidious. Adjacent organs may be affected by the inflammatory process, e.g. sympathetic pleural effusions. Pancreatic fluid collections following acute pancreatitis can include pseudocyst, pancreatic abscess, pancreatic necrosis, or infected necrosis. The following are more specific complications, which may occur in both acute and chronic pancreatitis.

PSEUDOCYST

This involves collection of pancreatic juice enclosed by fibrous tissue, either within or without the pancreas, but in any case beyond the normal pancreatic duct system. Pseudocysts develop in 25% of patients with chronic pancreatitis and in 10% with acute pancreatitis. They are more common in the body than in the head or tail of the pancreas.

Symptoms

Symptoms include pain, early satiety, or gastric outlet obstruction. Pancreatic pseudocysts may rupture, bleed, produce ascites, obstruct bile flow, compress the inferior vena cava, erode into the mediastinum, or become infected. Chronic pseudocysts cause fewer complications. Pseudocysts >6 cm in size do not resolve spontaneously.

Diagnosis

Diagnosis is generally made by CT (**197**) or ultrasound. Infection can be introduced at ERCP (**198**). EUS (with diagnostic cyst aspiration and assay for pancreatic enzymes) is especially useful in the differentiation of pancreatic pseudocysts from cystic tumours.

Treatment

Persisting pseudocysts are treated by drainage. This depends on local expertise, and may be by CT-guided percutaneous drainage (90% success), by EUS drainage into the stomach, or by surgical excision and internal or external drainage.

PANCREATIC INFECTION

Significant necrosis, as in acute pancreatitis, predisposes to infection. Recurrence of pain, fever, leukocytosis, or bacteraemia within 1–2 weeks of acute pancreatitis is often a presenting manifestation. Indolent abscesses may present after several weeks.

Diagnosis requires guided-needle aspiration, Gram stain, and culture. The wall is thicker and less well defined than in a pseudocyst.

Treatment requires prompt institution of broad-spectrum antibiotics. Surgical debridement may also be necessary.

Mortality ranges from 15–100%, depending upon promptness in diagnosis, aggressive treatment, identification of infectious organisms, and antibiotic susceptibility, as well as upon host factors.

SPLENIC VEIN THROMBOSIS

In coursing along the posterior surface of the pancreas, the splenic vein can be thrombosed due to peripancreatic oedema, inflammation, or seepage. Splenic vein thrombosis is five times

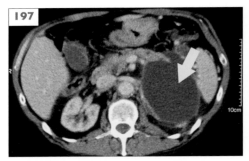

197 CT scan showing a large pseudocyst (arrowed) in the tail of the pancreas in a swollen, oedematous pancreas.

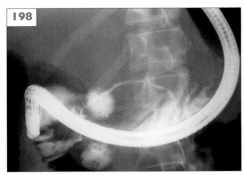

198 In addition to the pancreatic duct, there are cysts shown in connection with the duct.

more common in chronic than in acute pancreatitis. The condition causes extrahepatic portal hypertension, splenomegaly, and gastric varices.

Diagnosis is by Doppler ultrasound, CT or occasionally coeliac angiography. Splenectomy cures gastric varices.

PANCREATIC ASCITES

Pancreatic secretions (**190**) may enter the peritoneal cavity during acute as well as chronic pancreatitis. The ascites is characterized by elevated total protein, serum albumin, and pancreatic enzyme content. Coexisting pseudocysts are found in 60% of cases. Pancreatic ascites may develop in 15% of patients with chronic pancreatitis.

Most patients require surgery. ERCP may help to localize the pancreatic leak; stenting may be required.

PANCREATIC FISTULA

External fistulae are rare. Most are internal and occur after drainage or rupture of a pseudocyst, trauma, and surgery. The draining fluid is enriched in amylase. Diagnosis is by ERCP or a fistulogram. Management is usually conservative. Stenting of the duct, the use of the long-acting somatostatin analogue octreotide (to suppress pancreatic secretion), or surgery may be necessary.

Pancreatic tumours

ENDOCRINE PANCREATIC TUMOURS
Definition
These are tumours arising from the neuroendocrine system, which share characteristics of amine precursor uptake and decarboxylation (APUD)-omas.

Epidemiology and aetiology
Endocrine pancreatic tumours are uncommon, with a prevalence estimated at <10 cases per million of the population. In the majority of cases, they produce peptides. If secreted, these peptides give rise to distinctive clinical syndromes.

Gastrinoma and insulinoma are the most frequent endocrine pancreatic tumours (1–3 cases per million per year), compared with all other tumour types (<0.2 cases per million per year), which include glucagonoma, somatostatinoma, vasoactive intestinal peptide (VIP)-oma, growth hormone-releasing factor (GRF)-oma, and pancreatic polypeptide (PP)-oma. Nonfunctioning neuroendocrine tumours are more frequent (1% of all tumours found at autopsy, 36% of pancreatic endocrine tumours). Tumours may be sporadic or part of the MEN 1 syndrome, an autosomal dominant disorder affecting the *MEN1* gene on chromosome 11, with parathyroid, pancreas, and pituitary tumours.

Pathophysiology and pathology
Typically, endocrine pancreatic tumours appear as monotonous sheets of small, round cells with uniform nuclei and cytoplasm. Mitotic figures are few, consistent with the slow-growing nature of the tumours. Electron microscopy shows granules containing peptide hormones and other characteristic substances (e.g. amines, neurone-specific enolase, chromogranin). Tumours may produce more than one hormone. Histological typing does not predict the tumour growth pattern; malignant behaviour is more likely in tumours with necrosis, higher mitotic rates, and angioinvasion. The diagnosis of malignancy requires evidence for invasion of adjacent organs, lymph nodes, liver (**199**), or blood vessels. Only 5–10% of insulinomas are malignant, compared with 50–90% of other tumour types. The size of the tumours correlates with the malignancy potential. Similar endocrine tumours may be found in the lungs, jejunum, duodenum, or elsewhere.

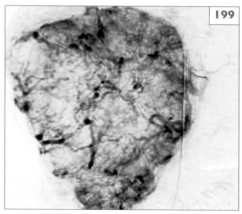

199 Hepatic angiogram in a neuroendocrine tumour of the liver showing massive hypervascular deposits.

History and physical findings

Manifestations depend upon the specific peptide produced by the tumours.

Gastrinoma

Typically, recurrent duodenal ulceration, diarrhoea, and hypergastrinaemia constitute the Zollinger–Ellison syndrome (see Chapter 4).

Insulinoma

Excess insulin release produces recurrent fasting hypoglycaemia, weight gain in a subconscious effort to avoid hypoglycaemia, psychiatric manifestations, palpitations, dizziness, and sweating.

VIPoma

Patients present with watery secretory diarrhoea, hypokalaemia, achlorhydria (WDHA syndrome, Verner–Morrison syndrome) and occasionally hyperglycaemia, hypercalcaemia, or flushing.

Glucagonoma

Patients with glucagonoma (**200**) present with migratory erythema (annular erythema affecting the buttocks, groin, perineum, or thighs, superficial bullae, erosions with crusting and hyperpigmentation), cheilitis, alopecia, and nail dystrophy. Glucose intolerance, anaemia, weight loss, diarrhoea, hypoaminoacidaemia, thromboembolism, and occasionally psychiatric manifestations and elevated ESR also occur.

Somatostatinoma

Patients present with hyperglycaemia, gallbladder disease, diarrhoea or steatorrhoea, hypochlorhydria, and weight loss.

GRFoma

Acromegaly is characteristic but may not be seen in all patients. Abdominal complaints related to hepatic metastases may be prominent. GRFoma is often associated with Zollinger–Ellison syndrome or MEN 1.

PPoma and nonfunctioning tumours

There are no specific symptoms related to peptide release. Cachexia, abdominal pain, hepatomegaly, gastrointestinal hypermotility, decreased gastric acid production, or exocrine pancreatic secretion may be present.

Other tumours

Symptoms include Cushing's syndrome due to corticotrophin release, and hypercalcaemia due to increased parathyroid hormone related protein.

Laboratory and special examinations

Diagnosis requires gut hormone assays to identify increased plasma levels of specific peptides, functional studies to demonstrate physiological consequences of peptide excess, and imaging studies to demonstrate the presence of tumours. In addition to specific hormones and biogenic amines, many endocrine pancreatic tumours secrete chromogranin A, which can be used in diagnosis as a nonspecific serum marker, and to track response to treatment. The primary tumour can be small and therefore difficult to localize. Various modalities include ultrasound (sensitivity 10–40%), CT (sensitivity 17–40%), EUS (sensitivity >80%), selective coeliac angiography (sensitivity 35–90%), multiple venous sampling for peptide assays, MRI (25–100% sensitivity), and intraoperative ultrasound (sensitivity >90%). Apart from insulinomas, many pancreatic endocrine tumours express type 2 somatostatin receptors, and can be detected and monitored with somatostatin-receptor scintigraphy.

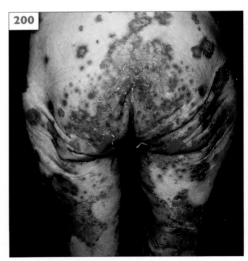

200 The characteristic rash in a patient with a glucagonoma.

Differential diagnosis
Neuroendocrine tumours simulate many common disorders, and a reasoned approach is essential.

Prognosis
The 5- to 10-year survival rates are >90% when no tumour is found (and by implication the tumour is very small) or when the tumour can be completely resected at surgery; rates are 15–75% with incomplete tumour resection or recurrent tumour; and 20–75% with unresectable tumours.

Management
Medical management may require the use of either specific peptide antagonists or symptomatic treatments to control metabolic abnormalities. Somatostatin analogues are useful in treating manifestations of VIPoma, as well as glucagonoma. Proton pump inhibitors at high dose are essential in gastrinoma (Zollinger–Ellison syndrome), to prevent gastroduodenal acid-mediated damage. Surgical outcomes improve with greater experience in tertiary referral centres. Chemotherapy is used for metastatic endocrine tumours. Debulking surgery may be undertaken. Symptomatic hepatic metastases may be treated by hepatic artery embolization. Orthotopic liver transplantation may improve survival in a small number of highly selected patients.

EXOCRINE PANCREATIC TUMOURS

Definition
An exocrine pancreatic tumour is a primary adenocarcinoma originating in pancreatic cells (excluding endocrine elements).

Epidemiology and aetiology
Tumours may originate from pancreatic ducts (88%), acinar cells (1%), connective tissue (0.6%), or mixed cell types (0.2%), or may be of uncertain or unclassified histogenesis (9%). The incidence of pancreatic adenocarcinoma (ductal origin) has risen to 11–12 per 100,000 of the population. The most affected age group is 60–80 years (80%) and the disease is uncommon in those younger than 40 years. The prevalence is greater in chronic pancreatitis (>nine-fold increase), diabetics (two- to three-fold increase), chronic smokers (approximately two-fold increase), urban populations, and after exposure to industrial carcinogens. Families with hereditary pancreatitis are at higher risk. These familial pancreatic cancer kindreds and Peutz–Jeghers patients should be screened.

Pathophysiology and pathology
The precise role of specific risk factors is unknown. There are well-differentiated, duct-like glands embedded in a dense matrix of fibrous tissue. Most pancreatic adenocarcinomas produce mucin (75%) and are located in the head of the pancreas. The tumours frequently extend to the retroperitoneum or invade adjacent organs, such as the stomach, duodenum, or gallbladder. Distant metastases are more frequently noted, with tumours arising in the body or tail of the pancreas.

Clinical history
Symptoms depend upon the location of the tumour. Neuropsychiatric manifestations, including depression and emotional lability, may be noted. Pruritus may be persistent.

Ampullary
Lesions affecting the ampulla of Vater present early with obstructive jaundice.

Pancreatic head
Tumours in the head of the pancreas may present with biliary or, more rarely, duodenal obstruction.

Pancreatic body and tail
Tumours arising in the body and tail tend to be 'silent' and therefore larger when they eventually become symptomatic. Poorly localized abdominal pain, anorexia, fatigue, and weight loss are frequent.

Physical examination
Hepatomegaly and jaundice are noted in 80% of cases, palpable gallbladder in 30% with carcinoma of the head of the pancreas, and abdominal mass, ascites, and oedema in 20%.

Laboratory and special examinations
Serum alkaline phosphatase, bilirubin, or blood sugar may be elevated. Plain radiograph of the abdomen may show the calcification of chronic pancreatitis. Pancreatic adenocarcinoma itself almost never calcifies. 'Sunburst' calcification is characteristic of benign cystadenoma.

A cavernous lymphangioma of pancreas may also calcify. Circulating antigens, including carcinoembryonic antigen (CEA), CA 19-9, and CA 125, are frequently raised, but have no diagnostic role by themselves, because they may be elevated in inflammatory disease.

Diagnosis and staging

Imaging studies are most helpful (**201–203**). The diagnostic approach is influenced by the likelihood of surgical resection. In patients unfit for major pancreatic resection, the diagnosis is frequently with transabdominal ultrasound or CT (sensitivity and specificity 80%). ERCP has sensitivity and specificity of 90%, and offers the opportunity for palliation in those with obstructive jaundice.

EUS- or CT-guided fine needle aspiration biopsy provides a tissue diagnosis in up to 90% of cases. EUS – with fine needle aspiration biopsy – is very sensitive, and will help in tumour staging and selecting patients for surgery. Complication rates for EUS-guided biopsy are lower than for percutaneous biopsy. Vascular invasion (superior mesenteric/portal vein) and relationship to regional arteries are key determinants of resectability and can be assessed by EUS. Coeliac angiography, although not usually required, is highly specific for vascular involvement, but is not very sensitive for diagnosis. Laparoscopy identifies 85% of the nonresectable tumours.

Differential diagnosis

Differentiate from benign adenoma of the papilla of Vater and other pancreatic tumours.

Prognosis

Prognosis remains very poor, as most patients present with late-stage disease. Only 10% of tumours are resectable. Median survival after chemotherapy is less than 20 weeks.

Management

Surgery pancreatico-duodenectomy (Whipple's procedure) is attempted for resection, and has an operative mortality rate of 2–20%. Only a minority of patients is suitable for an attempt at curative resection, and the role of adjuvant chemoradiotherapy is still uncertain.

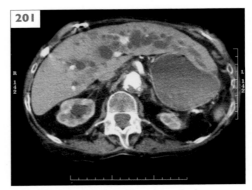

201 CT showing dilated intrahepatic ducts – there is biliary obstruction from an ampullary tumour.

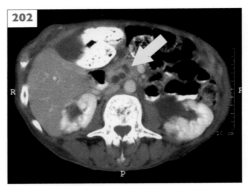

202 CT showing dilated pancreatic duct (arrowed).

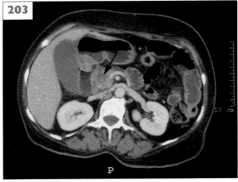

203 CT showing a mass in the head of pancreas.

Palliation

For the majority of patients, management is directed towards palliation rather than cure. Palliative surgery may be necessary for biliary or gastrointestinal obstruction (**204**). Chemotherapy with gemcitabine is usually considered. Gemcitabine is well tolerated, and so palliative chemotherapy can be appropriate even for frail patients. For jaundiced patients unsuitable for surgical resection, the mainstay of treatment is stenting the bile duct to relieve the obstruction. This may be done at ERCP or percutaneously under radiological guidance (**205**). Recurrent stent obstruction requiring stent changes is a frequent complication – self-expanding metallic stents remain patent for longer than plastic stents, but are more expensive (**206**). Pain relief is problematic and usually requires narcotic analgesics or coeliac axis neuronolysis by EUS, with percutaneous or CT guidance as appropriate. Exocrine pancreatic insufficiency may require pancreatic enzyme replacement.

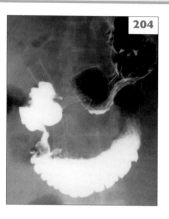

204 Barium meal showing duodenal obstruction from head of pancreas tumour (a metal stent is seen in the bile duct).

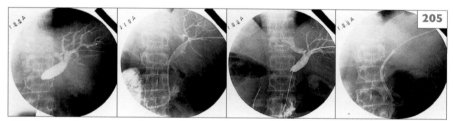

205 Pancreatic cancer causing extrahepatic obstruction. This is being relieved by the passage of a guidewire and dilatation. Subsequently, a permanent stent can be left *in situ*.

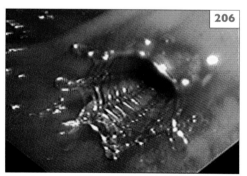

206 An expandable stent, seen from the duodenum, emerging from the bile duct where it is stenting an obstruction due to carcinoma of the pancreas.

Cystic lesions of the pancreas and other pancreatic neoplasms

There are a number of conditions presenting with cystic pancreatic lesions. Differentiating these is important, as some represent malignant and premalignant disease.

Retention cysts

These are small fluid-filled developmental cysts, lined by normal pancreatic tissue. They are rare and of no consequence.

Pseudocysts

These arise in the context of acute or chronic pancreatic inflammation, usually communicate with the pancreatic ducts, and contain pancreatic enzymes (see above).

Cystic neoplasms

There are a number of types of cystic neoplasms (**207–210**):

- Serous cystadenomas are typically comprised of multiple small cysts and are rarely malignant. Often there is a central scar – sometimes calcified. Serous cystadenomas are benign and usually asymptomatic.
- Mucinous cystic neoplasms (mucinous cystadenoma and mucinous cystadencarcinoma) are most frequent in middle-aged women. All have the potential for malignant change and are frequently malignant at diagnosis. They can be misinterpreted as pancreatic pseudocysts. However, unlike pseudocysts, mucinous cystic neoplasms have low amylase content, since they do not communicate with the pancreatic ducts.
- Intraductal papillary mucinous neoplasms are localized or diffuse lesions arising in the ducts, sometimes in chronic pancreatitis. They are most frequent in men, and produce thick, viscous mucin-rich secretion, which can block the pancreatic ducts and may emerge at the papilla.

Management

Most cystic lesions will have been detected by CT, ultrasound or some other cross-sectional imaging. Cysts should undergo aspiration/biopsy percutaneously or by EUS, with analysis of cyst contents for mucin (mucinous cystic neoplasms), glycogen-rich cells (suggestive of serous cystadenomas), and tumour markers such as CEA and CA 19-9. Mucinous cystic neoplasms, because of the potential for malignancy, are generally managed by surgical resection.

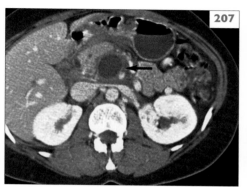

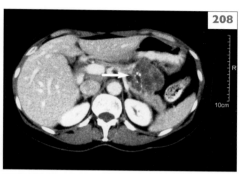

207 CT showing a cystic lesion in the body of pancreas (arrow).

208 CT showing multiple small cysts and central calcification. This 'bunch of grapes' appearance is most suggestive of serous cystadenoma (arrow).

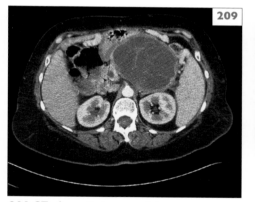

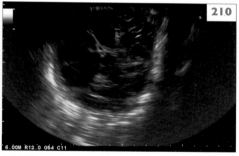

210 This is the same lesion as **209** – here seen at EUS. Fine needle aspiration showed this to be a mucinous tumour.

209 CT of a cystic tumour of the pancreas.

Biliary conditions

In the West, gallstones are the commonest cause of biliary symptomatology

Ultrasound (transabdominal and endoscopic) is the mainstay of diagnosis

Obstructive jaundice merits rapid investigation, and of itself can predispose to infection in the biliary tract

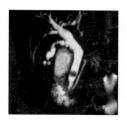
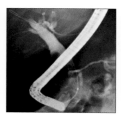
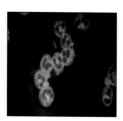
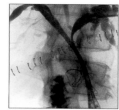

Anatomy

Intrahepatic bile ducts merge into main left and right hepatic ducts to form the common hepatic duct. This becomes the common bile duct below the origin of the cystic duct, which leads into the gallbladder. Bile flow from the liver is held temporarily in the gallbladder, but passes back into the common bile duct and hence the duodenum after eating. As with other tubular organs, mucosa, submucosa and muscle layers are present.

Investigations

Biliary conditions are investigated in a number of ways.

Plain radiography
This is frequently requested for patients with acute abdominal pain. The majority of gallstones are radiolucent, and so are not seen on plain X-ray, but some are radio-opaque (**211**). Gas in the biliary tree occurs in infection and following ampullary sphincterotomy.

Transabdominal ultrasound
This is the primary investigation of biliary disease. It is inexpensive, readily available, and noninvasive.

MRCP (synonym MR cholangiography)
This technique uses MR imaging to visualize the biliary tree. It has the advantage of being noninvasive, and so avoids the hazards of conventional ERCP. It is a purely diagnostic technique, but can be used in situations that are taxing or impossible for ERCP – for example, after Billroth II gastrectomy.

ERCP
MRCP is usurping the diagnostic role of ERCP. However, ERCP retains a major role in biliary interventions such as biopsy, extraction of gallstones from the bile duct, and placement of endobiliary stents – mainly for the palliation of biliary malignancy.

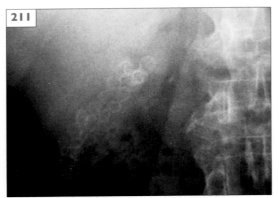

211 Calcified gallstones seen in this close-up of the right upper quadrant on plain abdominal X-ray.

Extrahepatic biliary disease

The hallmark is interference with bile flow due to stasis, obstruction, and/or infection. After secretion by hepatocytes into the bile canaliculi, bile is drained into enlarging ducts, which eventually lead to the gallbladder and the duodenum. Specialized epithelia lining the biliary passages serve secretory, as well as absorptive, functions. Common symptoms of biliary disease are jaundice, acute or recurrent upper abdominal pain, and fever with chills and rigors. Pathophysiologically distinct disorders include gallstone disease, benign or malignant biliary strictures, inflammatory conditions, parasitic infestations, congenital cysts, etc.

GALLSTONES
Definition
These are defined as stones arising in the gallbladder. Analogous stones also occur in intrahepatic and extrahepatic biliary ducts. Manifestations range from completely asymptomatic states to biliary obstruction, infection, and complications in other organs due to migration of stones. There is also an increased risk of gallbladder cancer.

Epidemiology and aetiology
Gallstones are among the most common disorders, and their prevalence has been rising. The incidence in people older than 40 years is approximately 3% per 5-year period. Cholesterol stones are most frequently encountered (75%). Gallstone formation is multifactorial and influenced by genetic-, age-, sex- and lifestyle-specific factors. Consequently, the overall prevalence varies significantly, being particularly high in Pima Indians, Caucasians in the United States, and Chileans, compared with Europeans or Asians. The aphorism for gallstones of 'fat, female, fertile, and forty' is not always true.

Pathophysiology
The most important elements are increased biliary cholesterol or pigment content, factors promoting nucleation of crystals, and gallbladder stasis. Diet and hepatic synthesis contribute to biliary cholesterol. Obesity, ageing, drugs, and hormones may increase biliary cholesterol secretion. Free cholesterol is insoluble, and bile acids and phospholipids are required for micelle formation. Deficiency of bile acid secretion or phospholipid production increases cholesterol saturation, when supersaturated cholesterol stones tend to form. Pigment stones may be 'black' or 'brown'. Black gallstones are smaller, amorphous, arise in patients with chronic haemolysis, and are frequently radio-opaque. Brown stones are found in the gallbladder and bile ducts, occur in the setting of cholangitis and infection, frequently recur, and are usually radiolucent.

Stone formation is aided by gallbladder stasis (for example during pregnancy or total parenteral nutrition), as well as by excess mucin. 'Biliary sludge' refers to microscopic precipitates of calcium bilirubinate, or cholesterol monohydrate crystals in mucin gels, which are visible on ultrasound. Gallstones are increased in conditions that promote biliary sludge.

History and physical examination
Approximately two-thirds of people with gallstones are asymptomatic. Nonspecific symptoms with indigestion, dyspepsia, flatulence, or intolerance to fatty foods are common. More specific manifestations produce characteristic symptoms.

Biliary colic
This occurs in 70–80% of symptomatic patients, due to transient cystic duct spasm or obstruction. Biliary colic pain may be precipitated by a large meal, is severe and episodic in nature, located in the epigastric or right and left upper abdominal regions, may radiate to the back or shoulder, and lasts for several hours (usually <6 hr).

Acute cholecystitis

Acute cholecystitis (**212**) is due to obstruction of the cystic duct (by gallstones in 90% of cases) Bacterial infection is usually secondary, but may produce gallbladder empyema. Acalculous acute cholecystitis occurs in 5–10% of patients in the setting of major surgery, critical illness, trauma, burns, and occasionally HIV infection or bone marrow transplantation. The pathophysiological events in acute cholecystitis include stasis, ischaemia, and necrosis. Pain lasting for >3 hr, and with local tenderness, vomiting, and fever is characteristic. Murphy's sign may be elicited (abrupt arrest in inspiration due to pain during abdominal palpation). In 30–40% of cases, a gallbladder and omental mass may be apparent; in 15% of cases, jaundice may appear. In the elderly, only localized tenderness may be seen.

Choledocholithiasis and cholangitis

These conditions arise when gallstones appear in the bile ducts. Small gallstones may pass unnoticed into the duodenum, whereas large stones are entrapped in the common bile duct. Common bile duct stones are often asymptomatic (45%) or present with complications, such as biliary colic, jaundice, cholangitis, and pancreatitis. Characteristic features of cholangitis are right upper quadrant pain, jaundice, chills, and rigor (Charcot's triad). Impaired bile flow gives rise to 'obstructive jaundice', with itching, clay-coloured stools, and biliary dilatation. In the setting of obstructive jaundice, a palpable gallbladder connotes malignancy. This is because gallstones induce chronic cholecystitis, and such a gallbladder is incapable of significant distension (Courvoisier's law). Unremitting biliary obstruction can produce secondary biliary cirrhosis within months.

Chronic cholecystitis

This is due to repeated episodes of apparent or inapparent gallbladder inflammation. Right upper quadrant pain of varying severity and frequency occurs. The presentation may be coloured by associated complications, such as

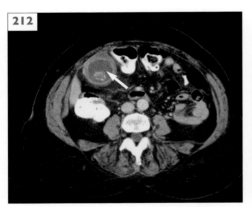

212 Acute cholecystitis. CT showing inflamed and oedematous gallbladder and gallstone.

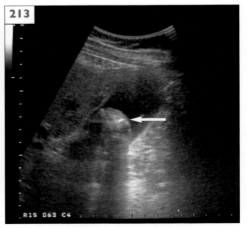

213 Ultrasound appearances of a large stone in the gallbladder with an acoustic shadow behind.

pancreatitis, cholangitis, or choledo-cholithiasis.

Laboratory and special examinations
• Biliary colic may be associated with no changes in blood tests.
• Acute cholecystitis is associated with leukocytosis, left-sided shift in neutrophils, and mild increases in serum aminotransferases (approximately two- to three-fold normal) or alkaline phosphatase (approximately one- to two-fold normal).
• Biliary obstruction produces markedly elevated serum alkaline phosphatase and bilirubin levels (>70% conjugated), although obstruction due to stones is rarely complete.

Imaging the biliary tract
Plain abdominal radiographs visualize only a minority of gallstones (13–17%) (**211**).

Transabdominal ultrasound is highly effective (sensitivity >90%) and allows assessment of gallbladder wall thickening and sludge, intramural gas, perigallbladder fluid collection, biliary dilatation, and gallbladder emptying (**213**). Oral cholecystography has virtually been replaced by ultrasound. EUS is more sensitive than transabdominal scanning, and is now the gold standard for detecting bile duct stones and microlithiasis.

Radioisotope scanning with ^{99m}Tc-HIDA (hepatic iminodiacetic acid) helps to establish gallbladder function, particularly in acute cholecystitis. HIDA is normally taken up by the gallbladder, but, in acute cholecystitis (or other causes of cystic duct obstruction), there is no gallbladder uptake of HIDA.

MRI and CT (**212**) are helpful when ultrasound imaging is unsatisfactory, and MRI can give excellent noninvasive images of the biliary tree (**214**).

Therapeutic intervention is often combined with imaging. Percutaneous transhepatic cholangiography (PTC) (**215**) or endoscopic

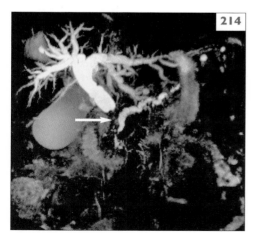

214 MRC showing short tight stricture in distal bile duct (arrow).

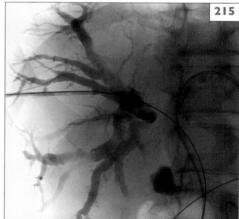

215 Carcinoma of common hepatic duct shown on PTC with multiple dilated ducts on the right side of the liver (compare with the MRC image shown in **214**).

retrograde cholangiography (ERC) (**216, 217**) can assess the biliary tree. The former is particularly easy when bile ducts are dilated. Therapeutic interventions may be combined with either PTC or ERC, including culture or cytology of bile, and insertion of draining stents.

Differential diagnosis

Other gallbladder disorders may mimic cholecystitis. These include cholesterolosis (cholesterol accumulation within histiocytes in gallbladder mucosa), adenoma, or adenomyomatous hyperplasia. Nonspecific abdominal symptoms require distinction from oesophagitis, acid peptic disease, gastrointestinal motility disorders, irritable colon syndrome, etc. Abdominal pain may be due to renal colic, appendicitis, pancreatitis, perforated peptic ulcer, intestinal obstruction, or other conditions. Lower-lobe pneumonia, pleural or pericardial disease, or coronary artery disease may also need to be considered.

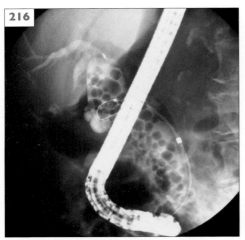

216 ERC showing a dilated common bile duct, containing multiple common duct stones.

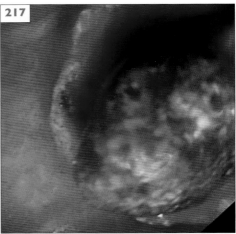

217 Gallstone trapped in bile duct being delivered into the duodenum at ERCP.

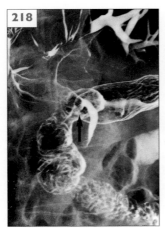

218 Choledocho-duodenal fistula from gallstones, demonstrated by barium meal – the barium is seen entering the bile duct and biliary tree through a fistula.

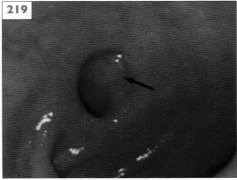

219 Appearance of the duodenum with a fistula leading into the bile duct, caused by prior passage of a stone (see 218).

Prognosis

Most gallstones are asymptomatic (60–80%). During a 20-year follow-up of patients, 50% remained asymptomatic, 30% developed biliary colic, and 20% manifested complications. The onset of biliary colic is associated with an increased risk of complications (particularly in the diabetic, elderly, or immunocompromised), such as cholangitis, pancreatitis, and gangrene or perforation of the gallbladder (10%). Acalculous disease has a poor prognosis, with a mortality rate of up to 70% in the presence of gallbladder gangrene, perforation, or empyema. Other complications include pericholecystic abscess, bile peritonitis, gallstone fistula (**218, 219**), and intestinal obstruction due to an impacted gallstone.

Management

Biliary colic is relieved with narcotic analgesics. Antibiotics active against Gram-negative microbes are necessary for treating cholangitis. Cholecystectomy is strongly advised for acute cholecystitis, as well as for chronic cholecystitis, unless there are medical contraindications, when antibiotics and intravenous (IV) fluid therapy may settle symptoms. Laparoscopic cholecystectomy is replacing open cholecystectomy because postoperative recovery is faster. Previous abdominal surgery, diffuse peritonitis, severe obesity, and pregnancy may limit laparoscopic cholecystectomy, however, and intraoperative bleeding or other intraoperative complications may warrant conversion to open surgery. Gallstone dissolution by oral bile acids is limited by frequent recurrence and requirement of <1.5 cm sized, noncalcified cholesterol stones within a functioning gallbladder.

Common bile duct stones may be diagnosed with EUS or MRCP (**220**). Most stones can be extracted at ERCP with the aid of an endoscopic papillotomy (**221**). In rare selected situations, gallstones may be dissolved by administering solvents, such as methyl terbutyl ether, via a T-tube placed surgically in the common bile duct, or a catheter placed percutaneously in the gallbladder. Extracorporeal shock wave lithotripsy has also been used to treat gallstones, although 20% of patients develop biliary colic and 10% develop pancreatitis during subsequent passage of the stone fragments.

Postcholecystectomy pain syndrome

In many individuals, pain or other symptoms persist after cholecystectomy. Mild diarrhoea due to an increased bile salt pool and bile salt spillage in the colon usually responds to cholestyramine. Recurrent abdominal pain (5% of cases) may be due to retained common bile duct stone, abscess, other surgical complications, or unrelated causes (such as irritable colon syndrome, peptic ulcer disease, pancreatitis, or biliary dyskinesia, which refers to delayed common bile duct emptying due to spasm in the sphincter of Oddi).

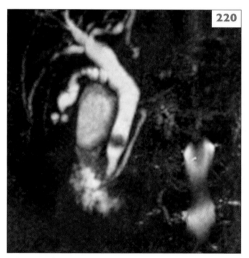

220 MRC showing gallstone in the common bile duct.

221 Same patient as 220 – pictures taken at ERCP when the stone was extracted.

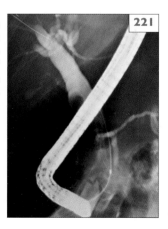

Choledochal cysts

Definition
These are congenital cystic malformations of the intra- or extrahepatic bile ducts. Several forms are recognized (**222**):
- Type 1: fusiform or saccular dilatation of the extrahepatic tree.
- Type 2: diverticular common bile duct cyst.
- Type 3: choledochocele.
- Type 4: diffuse dilatation of the common bile duct and hepatic ducts.
- Type 5: intrahepatic ductal dilatation (Caroli's disease).

Epidemiology and aetiology
No specific aetiology has been identified. The disorder is relatively infrequent. Most patients present in childhood, although up to 50% may present after the age of 10 years.

Pathophysiology
The cyst wall is thick, with dense connective tissue and smooth muscle. Pericystic inflammation may be noted, and cholangitis is a frequent complication. Compression of the common bile duct may cause obstructive jaundice and predispose to cholangitis.

Clinical history
This ranges from asymptomatic states to jaundice, abdominal pain, or fever in various combinations. Weight loss or failure to thrive may occur. Clay-coloured stools and pruritus may be prominent.

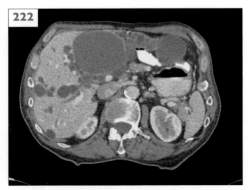

222 CT showing sacular and cyst-like dilatation of the intrahepatic biliary system in Caroli's disease.

Physical examination
Patients should be examined for jaundice, abdominal mass in the right upper quadrant, and upper abdominal tenderness.

Laboratory and special examinations
Mild to moderate increases in serum bilirubin and alkaline phosphatase are common. Manifestations of cholangitis or obstructive jaundice may be found. Transabdominal ultrasound, EUS, MR cholangiography, or CT all demonstrate dilated bile ducts or cystic lesions. ERC is most helpful for imaging the biliary tree and for typing.

Differential diagnosis
Distinction from biliary atresia in infants may be difficult, but is critical in establishing appropriate interventions. Other conditions include liver abscess, gallstones, and cancer.

Prognosis
Prognosis is usually excellent, although recurrent cholangitis may occur. Cholangiocarcinoma is more frequent in choledochal cysts.

Management
Treatment is surgical, although the specific operation depends upon the defect. It should always be considered because of the risk of malignancy. Simple cystenterostomy for biliary drainage might suffice. Complete cystectomy should be undertaken for choledochal cysts.

Gallbladder cancer

Epidemiology and aetiology
Gallbladder adenocarcinoma is relatively infrequent in the West and more common in the East. There is a 3:1 greater prevalence in women. Patients tend generally to be older (>70 years) and with coexisting gallstones (80–90%). The risk factors for gallstones and gallbladder carcinoma are the same. The incidence of gallbladder carcinoma is increased with very large gallstones (>3 cm), and with gallbladder calcification producing 'porcelain gallbladder' on plain radiographs or CT (**223**). In some cases, a precancerous neoplastic adenomatous polyp may have been identified (**224**).

Pathophysiology
Prolonged inflammation and increased epithelial cell turnover probably contribute to neoplastic

transformation, although genetic changes in gallbladder carcinoma are undefined.

Clinical history
Early manifestations may be nonspecific and complicated by coexisting gallstone disease. Persistent upper abdominal pain or unremitting jaundice may first indicate more serious disease. Anorexia, fatigue, and weight loss may be noted.

Physical examination
Jaundice and a vaguely defined firm or hard mass in the right upper quadrant are typical.

Laboratory and special examinations
Both conjugated and unconjugated hyperbilirubinaemia are present, due to a combination of biliary obstruction and hepatic dysfunction. Other manifestations may include low serum albumin, prolonged prothrombin time, and elevated serum alkaline phosphatase. Imaging will demonstrate gallbladder lesions (**225**, **226**), commonly accompanied by liver metastases. EUS may be helpful for staging, and fine needle aspiration biopsy can establish tissue diagnosis.

Differential diagnosis
Differentiate from other causes of obstructive or mixed cholestatic/hepatocellular-type jaundice.

Prognosis
Gallbladder carcinoma can be resected in <20% of cases. Disease commonly extends to the bile ducts, liver, and portal lymph nodes, as well as to distant organs. In the presence of jaundice, gallbladder carcinoma is unresectable in >85% of patients.

Management
Chemotherapy and radiotherapy are ineffective. Care is usually aimed at symptomatic palliation, including relief of biliary obstruction by internal stents.

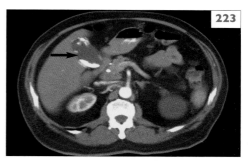

223 Porcelain gallbladder on CT scan. This is an uncommon manifestation of chronic cholecystitis.

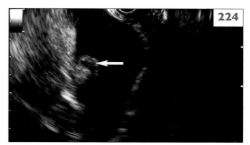

224 A large gallbladder polyp (nonmobile) is seen protruding from the gallbladder wall on the EUS image.

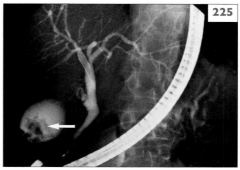

225 Mass in the fundus of the gallbladder.

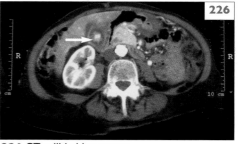

226 CT gallbladder cancer.

Primary sclerosing cholangitits

Definition
Primary sclerosing cholangitits (PSC) is an insidious and progressive inflammatory disorder, with immunological abnormalities resulting in fibrosis and segmental obliteration of large bile ducts.

Epidemiology and aetiology
The cause is unknown, but a strong association exists with inflammatory bowel disease. PSC occurs in approximately 3–5% of all patients with inflammatory bowel disease, while up to 50% of PSC patients may manifest with inflammatory bowel disease. If fully investigated to detect subclinical disease, 80–90% of PSC patients may be shown to have inflammatory bowel disease, and the proportion will rise with time. Inflammatory bowel disease is much more commonly ulcerative colitis than Crohn's disease, and occurs more frequently in men than in women; the mean age of diagnosis is 40 years. However, PSC does not remit after colectomy, and there is no correlation between disease activity of inflammatory bowel disease and PSC. The prevalence of HLA-B8 and DR3 is increased in PSC.

Pathophysiology
A variety of immunological abnormalities has been noted, but the precise significance of these observations remains unclear. Autoantibodies have been identified, directed against shared antigens displayed on colon and biliary epithelial cells. Liver biopsy early in the natural history demonstrates periportal accumulation of small and large lymphocytes, periductular inflammation and destruction, and 'onion-skin' liver fibrosis (**227**) through to cirrhosis late in the natural history (stage 4).

Clinical history
This ranges from insidious onset of chronic cholestasis to recurrent episodes of cholangitis (15–20% of cases). Pruritus, weight loss, fatigue, and malaise may be noted. An asymptomatic isolated increase in serum alkaline phosphatase levels may antedate symptoms by months to years.

Physical examination
The liver may be normal in size or mildly enlarged. Splenomegaly and ascites may develop in the late stages, due to portal hypertension.

Laboratory and special examinations
Biochemical parameters are indicative of cholangitis or cholestasis. Hypergammaglobulinaemia is common – especially IgM. A characteristic autoantibody (antineutrophil cytoplasmic antibody, ANCA) can generally be found in the circulation (**228**), but is not diagnostic. The diagnosis is best established by demonstration of characteristic morphological changes in bile ducts, preferably by MRCP, although ERCP (**229**, **230**), remains more sensitive for early disease. Liver biopsy may also be diagnostic and required to late-stage disease, or to differentiate from other cholestatic liver disorders.

Differential diagnosis
Differentiate from other cholestatic disorders, including primary biliary cirrhosis. Benign biliary strictures may arise from trauma, infection, ischaemia, and hepatic arterial chemotherapy. Recurrent infection in the setting of benign strictures can lead to secondary sclerosing cholangitis. Diffuse cholangiocarcinoma can give similar imaging appearances. Infectious cholangiopathy in the setting of AIDS (cryptosporidia or microsporidia) may need to be distinguished.

Small duct PSC
This is a variant of PSC, accounting for fewer than 5% of patients. It affects the smaller bile ducts – beyond the resolution of ERCP.

Prognosis
The most important prognostic indicators are age, serum bilirubin, liver histology, and the presence or absence of splenomegaly. If untreated, PSC patients demonstrate progressive deterioration over a prolonged period of 10–20 years, ultimately with hepatic failure. Cholangiocarcinoma is a frequent complication (20–30%).

Management
No specific therapies are available to treat PSC. Anti-inflammatory and antifibrotic therapies, including corticosteroids, azathioprine,

methotrexate, and others, have been used. However, none has been convincingly shown to alter the natural history of the disease, or to delay the interval to liver transplant. Ursodeoxycholic acid may improve pruritus, as well as biochemical parameters.

Management of complications

The mainstays are antibiotics for symptomatic bacterial cholangitis. Pruritus is a common and disabling symptom. It may respond to bile-binding agents such as cholestyramine, or enzyme-inducing drugs such as rifampicin.

'Dominant' strictures in the bile duct can be managed by endoscopic dilatation at ERCP. Distinctions between stricturing lesions and cholangiocarcinoma may be particularly difficult and require brush cytology, as well as biopsy.

Prolonged cholestasis may be accompanied by deficiencies of fat-soluble vitamins. Appropriate supplements, particularly to prevent bone disease, are necessary. Associated pancreatic insufficiency or coeliac disease, which can contribute to steatorrhoea, should be dealt with.

Orthotopic liver transplantation in advanced disease provides excellent outcomes.

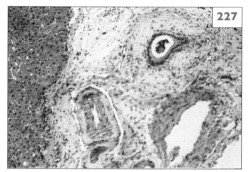

227 Liver biopsy appearances in sclerosing cholangitis, showing 'onion-skin' fibrosis around the bile ducts.

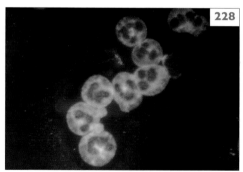

228 ANCA – an autoantibody in the serum of most patients with sclerosing cholangitis, detected by immunofluorescence on normal neutrophils.

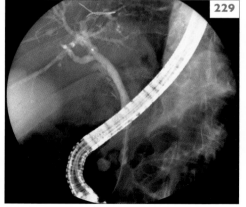

229 ERCP examination of the liver showing truncated irregular intrahepatic bile ducts in PSC.

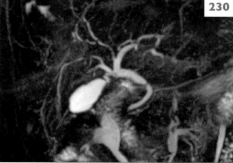

230 MRCP showing truncated and irregular bile ducts of PSC.

Cholangiocarcinoma

Definition
This is an adenocarcinoma originating in the biliary epithelium.

Epidemiology and aetiology
Overall, males are more frequently affected. Cholangiocarcinoma is more prevalent in the Far East, in the setting of cholangiohepatitis, and also complicates PSC (**231**) and choledochal cysts. The diagnosis of all biliary tract cancers is increasing, and this increase is not only because of better imaging.

Pathophysiology
Polypoid, sclerosing, or infiltrating tumours are present. Poorly defined thickening of the bile duct wall leads to luminal narrowing, often resembling fibrous strictures or sclerosing cholangitis. Tumours are slow-growing, with a tendency to infiltrate the duct wall and spread to the lymph nodes. The tumours may be intrahepatic (5–10%) or outside the liver, in the distal bile duct (20–25%), or most commonly at the hilum or the junction of the right and left hepatic bile ducts (60–70%).

Clinical history
Patients present with vague upper abdominal pain, an asymptomatic increase in serum alkaline phosphatase without jaundice, progressive obstructive jaundice, or cholangitis.

Physical examination
Patients should be examined for mild hepatomegaly in the presence of obstructive jaundice. Ill-defined upper abdominal masses may be present in the advanced stages.

Laboratory and special examinations
Biochemical findings are nonspecific, and consistent with partial or total biliary obstruction. Tumour markers (CEA and CA 19-9) are frequently raised, but are not specific.

Staging investigations
Distal bile duct lesions
These are staged with ultrasound, CT, or MRCP, followed by EUS with biopsy (**232**). Laparoscopy is reserved for staging potentially resectable disease (**233**). ERCP with a view to establishing biliary drainage is appropriate for patients unsuitable for curative surgery. ERCP also permits precise localization of the biliary abnormality, as well as cytology of the aspirated bile or brushings (**234**).

Proximal bile duct lesions
Proximal bile duct lesions are staged in a similar way to distal bile duct lesions. They can be suspected when ultrasound indicates intrahepatic duct dilatation, without dilatation of the extrahepatic system. Vascular involvement is critical to surgical planning, and EUS or MR imaging can assess hilar vascular invasion. A heterogeneous hepatic mass may be apparent on imaging. EUS with fine needle aspiration biopsy may be diagnostic. Laparoscopy is used to assess potential surgical candidates. Percutaneous cholangiography may sometimes be required to achieve biliary drainage, and is more likely to be successful than ERCP (**235**). Preoperative biliary drainage with decompression is appropriate if resection is contemplated; palliation of inoperable obstructive jaundice is required.

Differential diagnosis
Differentiate from benign biliary strictures, primary sclerosing cholangitis, pancreatic carcinoma, lesions of the ampulla of Vater, hepatocellular carcinoma, lymph node metastases in the porta hepatis, and other cholestatic disorders.

Management
Distal duct cholangiocarcinoma
Surgery is the only curative approach, although resection is usually not possible. Surgery for low bile duct lesions is pancreatico-duodenectomy, which is similar to that for head of pancreas cancer.

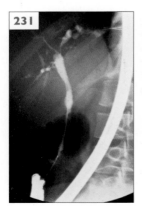

231

231
Cholangiocarcinoma complicating PSC – there is a stricture in the bile duct seen at ERCP.

Hilar lesions

Surgery involves extended liver resection. This is usually preceded by decompression of the obstructed hepatic segments. There are encouraging reports of surgery following elective portal vein embolization, to facilitate atrophy of the affected lobe and promote compensatory hypertrophy in the remaining liver prior to resection.

External beam radiotherapy

This is generally limited by toxicity to adjacent organs, although brachytherapy (intraductal radiation by implanted sources) shows some promise. Palliative chemotherapy is a further option. Orthotopic liver transplantation for intrahepatic cholangiocarcinoma has been very disappointing due to early recurrence.

Palliation of jaundice

Endobiliary stents can be placed at ERCP; metallic stents will remain patent longer than plastic stents. ERCP is less likely to succeed in stenting hilar and intrahepatic disease, for which PTC or a combined PTC and ERC approach is frequently required.

Prognosis

At laparotomy, only one-third of the tumours are resectable. The 5-year survival rate after attempted resection is approximately 20%. Most patients die of hepatic invasion and liver failure.

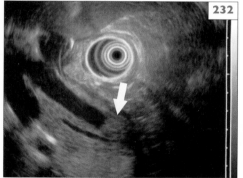

232 EUS image with a tumour in the distal bile duct (arrowed).

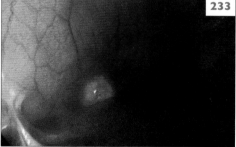

233 A peritoneal metastasis seen at laparoscopy. Laparoscopy is used to stage various upper gastrointestinal malignancies – here the primary was a cholangiocarcinoma.

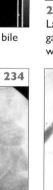

234 Cholangiocarcinoma of lower bile duct at ERCP – a stent being placed.

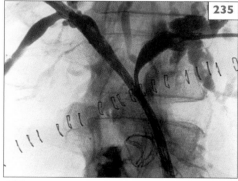

235 Multiple stents placed at PTC in patient with hilar cholangiocarcinoma.

Cholangiohepatitis

Definition
This is defined as recurrent episodes of cholangitis, due to intrahepatic bile duct stones, often in conjunction with parasitic infestation.

Epidemiology and aetiology
The condition is most frequently encountered in South East Asia (50–80%) and only rarely in Western countries (0.6–2.4%). Patients tend to be younger than those with gallbladder stones, from poor socioeconomic situations, and frequently suffer from malnutrition. Associated parasitic infestations include *Clonorchis sinensis* (25%) and ascariasis (13–20%). Gallbladder stones may coexist in 33% of the patients.

Pathophysiology
Parasites in intrahepatic bile ducts interfere with biliary drainage, induce recurrent episodes of cholangitis, and excite the host immune response with hepatic fibrosis, bile duct proliferation, dilatation, and suppuration. Black pigment stones containing calcium bilirubinate are frequent.

Clinical history
Recurrent pain, fever, and jaundice occurring at intervals of weeks, months, or years are typical.

Physical examination
Patients should be examined for jaundice, hepatomegaly (19% of cases), and a palpable gallbladder (9%).

Laboratory and special examinations
Plain radiograph of the abdomen is unhelpful. CT tends to be more helpful than ultrasound in demonstrating calcific lesions or hepatic abnormalities. ERCP and PTC are most helpful in diagnosis. Biliary strictures are frequent (35%), and most commonly involve the left hepatic duct (90%).

Differential diagnosis
Differentiate from other causes of cholangitis.

Prognosis
Prognosis depends upon the duration of symptoms, and the severity of biliary strictures and liver disease. Mortality rates within 4 weeks of surgical therapy approach 4–10%, and increase progressively with multiple surgical interventions. Acalculous cholecystitis (40% of cases) is often severe and may prove fatal.

Management
The mainstays are surgery and endoscopic intervention, the goals being to remove ductal stones, drain obstructed segments of the bile ducts, and dilate strictures. Eradication of parasites may not arrest or reverse disease.

Colonic disease

Colonic cancer is common. As there are generally many years of benign adenomatous growth before malignancy occurs, it is also preventable

Ulcerative colitis can present as a medical emergency and urgent treatment may avoid the need for colectomy

Colonoscopy and biopsy are the most effective diagnostic manoeuvres

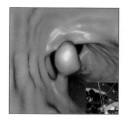
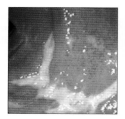
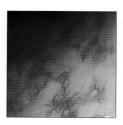
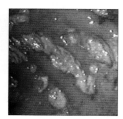

Anatomy

The colon is approximately 1.5 m long, commencing in the right iliac fossa at the ileocaecal valve. It consists of the caecum, ascending colon, transverse colon, descending colon, sigmoid colon, and rectum.

The transverse colon and sigmoid colon are particularly mobile on a free mesentery, while the caecum, ascending colon, and descending colon are relatively fixed without a free mesentery. The lower 12 cm of the rectum lie below the peritoneal reflection.

INVESTIGATIONS

The major investigations of the colon are radiological (contrast radiology with barium and CT) or endoscopic. The correct method of investigation varies, and will depend on local resources and availability. The procedures are complementary.

Barium enema

This is best performed after a few days on a low-residue diet, and emptying the colon by either laxatives or colonic lavage. Barium is run in, evacuated, and air insufflated, to give single and air-contrast barium enemas (**236**). The procedure should not be performed if there is active inflammatory bowel disease of more than mild severity.

Rigid sigmoidoscopy

This visualizes the lowest 12–28 cm of the bowel, and biopsies can be taken. No preparation is needed. The technique is useful for assessing the presence/activity of colitis.

Flexible sigmoidoscopy

This visualizes the left side of the colon; a simple enema to empty the colon is generally needed. It is useful for investigating some forms of rectal bleeding and for screening the left side of the colon for cancer, as most tumours/polyps are left-sided. The procedure is quicker and more convenient than full colonoscopy, but this is a compromise.

Colonoscopy

This aims to visualize the whole of the colon (unless the bowel is very tortuous, or there are deviations from the normal anatomy, **237–239**).

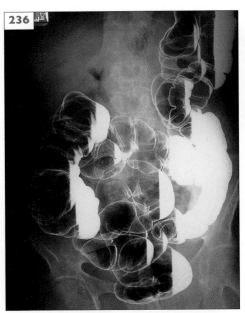

236 Normal barium enema (taken in the left lateral decubitus position), showing distinction between air contrast and barium contrast.

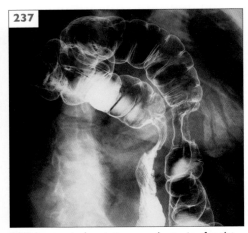

237 Anatomical variations can be taxing for the colonoscopist. In this barium enema, the colon is seen herniating into the chest through a congenital diaphragmatic hernia.

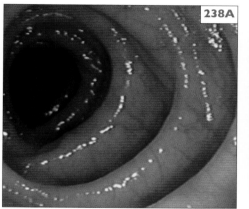

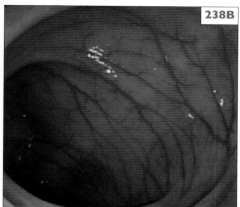

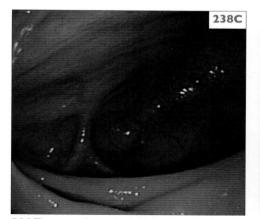

238 There are few reliable landmarks in colonoscopy. This figure illustrates: (**A**) the descending colon; (**B**) the dark organ seen through the colonic wall, suggesting that this is the splenic flexure; and (**C**) the lips of the ileocaecal valve.

239 Intubation into the ileum is often possible at colonoscopy − note the small-intestinal villi.

A full preparation to empty the bowel is required.

The advantage of both flexible sigmoidoscopy and colonoscopy is that multiple biopsies can be taken. Therapeutic procedures such as polypectomy can also be undertaken. Colonoscopy is much more sensitive than barium enema, which has an appreciable 'miss rate'.

New colonoscopic techniques increase sensitivity for detecting subtle lesions, and assist in targeting endoscopic biopsies of regions of interest. These include magnifying colonoscopes and confocal laser microscopy, which give endoscopic images similar to conventional histology. Enhancing mucosal contrast by 'chromoendoscopy' uses dye spraying of the mucosa to reveal the pit patterns of colonic polyps, and to facilitate distinction between adenomas and hyperplastic polyps. Narrow band imaging and multiband imaging utilize different wavelengths of light to improve the assessment of mucosal abnormalities.

CT scanning

This can be used to investigate the bowel. Protocols vary, but all require the patient to drink a contrast agent to outline the luminal surface of the bowel (**240**).

CT colography (synonym virtual colonoscopy)

This is a specialized CT technique to evaluate the colon. Following full bowel preparation, the patient is scanned prone and supine. Dedicated software is used to reconstruct the CT images of the bowel, which are very reminiscent of a physical colonoscopy (**241**). Depending on the enthusiasm and expertise of the radiologist, CT colograms are able to resolve smaller and smaller colonic polyps. The resolution will continue to improve, as the technology is refined.

Other investigations

- Plain X-ray (**242**) – displays the presence or absence of colonic dilatation, obstruction, and volvulus, and is often helpful in delineating the extent of inflammatory colitis.

- Labelled leukocyte scanning – identifies areas of inflammation (e.g. ulcerative colitis, Crohn's disease, pseudomembranous colitis).
- Anorectal manometry – for the investigation of incontinence or severe constipation.

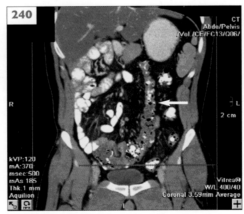

240 CT of the large bowel – this view taken from a 3D reconstruction illustrates partial malrotation of the large bowel. (The ascending colon is left of the midline, and the small bowel in the right upper quadrant.)

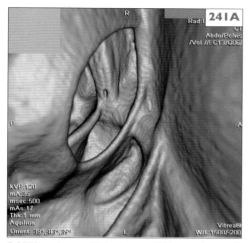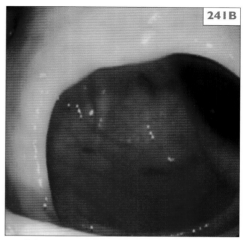

241 View from a CT cologram (**A**), together with view of the caecum in the same patient from colonoscopy (**B**).

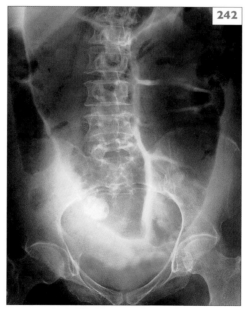

242 Sigmoid volvulus showing grossly dilated colon extending from the left of the pelvis and giving a typical 'coffee bean' appearance.

Colonic polyps

Definition
Polyps are abnormal structures that arise from the gastrointestinal mucosa and protrude into the lumen. Colonic polyps may be single or multiple, sessile or pedunculated, and sporadic or hereditary in origin.

Epidemiology and aetiology
The origin of colonic polyps is multifactorial. Several histological types are recognized.

Hyperplastic polyps
These are characterized by metaplastic change, but have no neoplastic potential. Hyperplastic polyps are small, asymptomatic, and are usually found at endoscopy undertaken for other reasons. They are mostly located in the rectum and distal sigmoid colon, and are frequent (20% of all polyps). Rare hyperplastic polyposis syndromes are associated with either more than 30 polyps, or proximal and larger hyperplastic polyps.

Inflammatory polyps
These are also non-neoplastic and arise in the setting of chronic mucosal inflammation, e.g. ulcerative colitis. They are restricted to areas of the inflamed bowel.

Juvenile polyps
These are hamartomas of the lamina propria, may be single or multiple, are mostly situated in the rectum, and may present with haemorrhage or autoamputation.

Adenomatous polyps
These are neoplastic, and thus of the greatest concern. The incidence of adenomatous polyps increases with age and parallels the risk for colon carcinoma. In the United States, adenomatous polyps are present in 40–50% of people aged over 60 years. In contrast, they are infrequent in populations at low risk for colon carcinoma, e.g. in black South Africans (<0.5%) or the Japanese (10%). The risk of colon carcinoma in patients with adenomatous polyps is related to the polyp size, and not to the number of polyps.

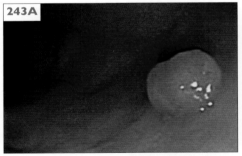

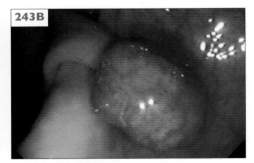

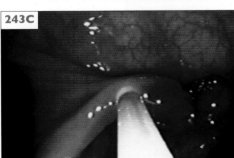

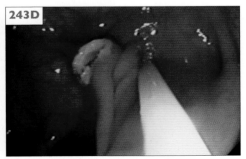

243 Colonic polyps. Polyps have a variety of forms: (**A**) small sessile polyp; (**B**) pedunculated polyp; (**C**) the polyp being snared; and (**D**) the resected polyp stalk.

Adenomatous polyps may be tubular (60%; small, spherical, stalk present, lobulated surface), villous (10%; large, sessile, velvety surface with fronds), or tubulovillous (30%; hybrid features). Adenomatous polyps display dysplastic changes with nuclear abnormalities, as well as a glandular architecture. Several genetic disorders are recognized with specific chromosomal abnormalities leading to adenomatous polyps (see p. 167).

Flat adenomas and serrated polyps
Not all polyps project as a protuberance into the colonic lumen. Flat adenomas and serrated polyps form the minority of colonic polyps. Flat adenomatous polyps are harder to detect (e.g. with CT colography), and their role in colorectal carcinogenesis is less well understood.

Pathophysiology
The colonic epithelium is normally replenished every 3–8 days, with migration of proliferating cells from the bottom of the mucosal crypts toward the surface. In adenomas, cellular DNA synthesis is amplified, immature epithelial cells are found in the crypts closer to the mucosal surface, and proliferating cells accumulate on the luminal surface, producing new adenomatous tissues. The relationship between adenomatous polyps and colon carcinoma was deduced from their similar epidemiological features and anatomical distributions, the presence of adenomatous tissue in small cancers, adenoma–carcinoma transition in familial polyposis syndromes, decreased risk of colon cancer after removal of polyps, and a lag period of several years between the onset of polyps and progression to malignancy.

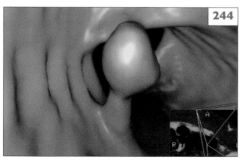

244 Polyp seen on CT cologram – similar to the view at colonoscopy.

Clinical history
Most colonic polyps are asymptomatic. Occult blood in the stool is frequent. Rectal bleeding is occasionally reported with large polyps.

Physical examination
Polyps may sometimes be palpable on rectal examination. Screening sigmoidoscopy may demonstrate silent polyps, and usually colonoscopy is recommended if multiple polyps, a large polyp, or tubulovillous polyps are found.

Laboratory and special examinations
A blood count and iron studies may unmask iron-deficiency anaemia. Polyps may be demonstrated by double-contrast barium enema (sensitivity 80–90%). Colonoscopy is more sensitive (up to 98%) and provides the added advantage of biopsy or removal of the polyps; thus, it remains the gold standard. CT colography is not yet a mature technology, but it is becoming increasingly sensitive to the presence of small polyps (**243, 244**). It is less invasive than physical colonoscopy and has the potential advantage of identifying polyps 'hidden' behind mucosal folds, which can be overlooked by conventional colonoscopy.

Differential diagnosis
It is crucial to differentiate between various types of polyps and colon cancer.

Prognosis
Colon carcinoma occurs in 1–3%, 10%, and 40% of polyps with sizes of <1 cm, 1–2 cm, and >2 cm, respectively. Polyps with villous architecture are most frequently malignant (40%), followed by tubulovillous (23%) and tubular (<5%) polyps. Adenomatous polyps have a tendency to recur and prolonged surveillance is required. The prognosis is worse in the presence of poorly differentiated polyps, penetration of muscularis mucosae, vascular or lymphatic invasion, and cancer in the resection margin.

Management
Most colonic polyps are removed or destroyed by endoscopic procedures, such as a 'hot biopsy' or snare diathermy, using electrocautery. Surgery is only rarely necessary. As new adenomatous polyps tend to develop, colonoscopy is performed 1 year after polyp removal and, when no further polyps are found, at 3- to 5-year intervals.

Colon carcinoma

Definition
Colon carcinoma is an adenocarcinoma originating in the large intestine and rectum.

Epidemiology and aetiology
Colon carcinoma is frequent in North America, north-western Europe, and New Zealand, but less common in South America, South East Asia, equatorial Africa and India. The incidence increases in people after migration from low- to high-incidence areas.

Genetic factors
The genetic mechanisms include chromosomes 17 and 18, with the 'deleted in colon carcinoma (DCC)' gene and the 'nucleotide mismatch repair' genes, as well as proto-oncogene abnormalities, such as in the *c-myc*, *c-Ki-ras* and *p53* genes. The nucleotide mismatch repair gene abnormalities are transmitted as autosomal dominant with a high penetrance, as in hereditary nonpolyposis colorectal cancer (HNPCC).

Risk factors
Low intake of dietary fibre, calcium, or vitamin D, excess consumption of saturated animal fats, and obesity increase risk, whereas high consumption of anticarcinogens in fruits and vegetables may decrease risk. Intake of aspirin and NSAIDs appears to protect against colon cancer. Other risk factors are age over 50 years, long-standing ulcerative colitis or Crohn's disease, past history of colon adenoma or cancer, breast cancer and female genital tract cancer (Lynch II syndrome), and family history of polyposis syndromes or colorectal carcinoma.

Pathophysiology
Colonic adenocarcinoma most commonly follows the polyp–adenoma–carcinoma sequence, involving uncontrolled cell proliferation in the epithelial crypts. There is varying glandular differentiation and mucin production. Right-sided colonic tumours are more frequently polypoid, and left-sided tumours annular or constricting. The distal 60 cm of the colon harbours 50% of the tumours. The descending colon, sigmoid colon, and rectum contain most tumours (75%), followed by the caecum and ascending colon (15%), and the transverse colon (10%). Tumours spread by direct extension into pericolonic fat, mesentery, surrounding organs, and peritoneal cavity, by lymphatics to the lymph nodes, and via the portal vein to the liver.

Clinical history
Rectal bleeding, change in bowel habit, colonic obstruction, and iron-deficiency anaemia are all common presentations. Right-sided tumours are more likely to present with anaemia, left-sided with frank bleeding or obstruction. Pedigree analysis is helpful when appropriate.

Physical examination
A rectal mass may be digitally palpated. Signs of liver disease, localized perforation, peritonitis, and abdominal masses may be noted. Manifestations may be of distant metastases; around one-third of patients present with metastatic disease.

Laboratory and special examinations
Biochemical and haematological tests are nondiagnostic. Serum CEA is of no value in screening.

Endoscopic tests include:
- Flexible sigmoidoscopy plus double-contrast barium enema – often adequate (**245**).
- Colonoscopy – necessary for tissue diagnosis of lesions proximal to the descending colon (**246**).
- Imaging modalities – thoracoabdominal and pelvic CT, endoanal EUS, and MRI (of the rectum, **247**), used for tumour staging.

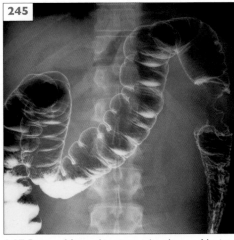

245 Barium X-ray showing an 'apple core' lesion in the descending colon.

Differential diagnosis

Differentiate from carcinoma of the anal canal (lymphoma, leiomyosarcoma, malignant carcinoid, Kaposi's sarcoma). Differentiate also from invasion of cancers from adjacent organs (prostate, ovary, uterus, or stomach). Benign lesions that may mimic colonic cancer include benign polyps, lipoma of the ileocaecal valve, and others.

Prognosis

The 10-year survival rate after resection approaches 40%. Survival is dependent upon tumour staging (Dukes' classification and TNM classification are both used).

Dukes' class A (confined to mucosa), B (extending through all areas of bowel wall), and C (regional lymph nodes) are associated with 5-year survival rates of 80–90%, 70–80%, and 30–55%, respectively; 80% of metastatic disease is manifest within 3 years of surgery.

The TNM stages O (*in situ* cancer), I (limited to the mucosa, submucosa, or external muscle), II (penetration of all adjacent bowel layers), III (spread to regional lymph nodes, nearby tissues, or organs), and IV (distant sites, e.g. liver, lungs) are associated with generally similar outcomes.

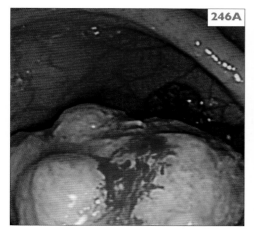

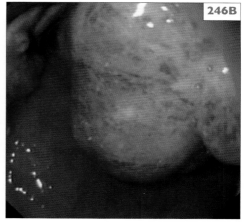

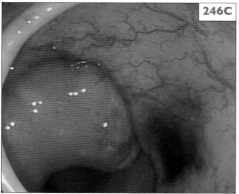

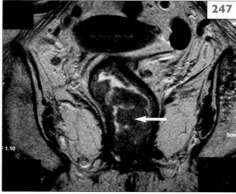

246 Colonic cancer – the endoscopic views (**A, B**) show various polypoid forms. In (**C**), the lesion has been 'tattooed' by the endoscopist to help the surgeon locate the tumour at laparoscopy.

247 MRI scan (in coronal section) showing bulky rectal tumour.

Management

A multidisciplinary approach is essential in planning treatment.

Localized disease

Surgical resection with curative intent should be offered to suitable patients with localized disease (**248**). The guiding surgical principles are to remove the affected segment, omentum, and draining lymph nodes. A hemicolectomy is necessary for right- or left-sided lesions. Lesions in the sigmoid colon and rectum are resected with wide margins.

Adjuvant chemotherapy with fluorouracil and the oral agent capecitabine have shown survival benefit in patients with Dukes' C disease and patients with 'high-risk' Dukes' B disease.

Rectal disease

Short-course radiotherapy (five fractions) has shown a benefit in overall survival, as well as in local control. Patients with bulky disease, in whom MRI suggests compromise of the mesorectal margin, should be considered for long-course chemoradiation. Postoperative radiotherapy is given to patients who have not had preoperative radiotherapy, if the tumour involves, or is close, to the resection margin.

Advanced disease

Solitary hepatic metastases may be amenable to surgical resection after the primary lesion is resected. Liver metastases are found in 50% of those with advanced disease. In the many patients who present with advanced disease, only palliative therapy may be practical – for example, decompressive colostomy, or endoscopic therapy such as laser photoablation or colonic stenting to relieve colonic obstruction. Palliative chemotherapy has an important role, with an increase in the number of drugs available over recent years. Fluorouracil, including its oral counterparts, is often used in conjunction with oxaliplatin or irinotecan.

Biological agents, including vascular endothelial growth factor (VEGF) and epidermal growth factor receptor (EGFR) inhibitors, also show promise.

Anal cancer

Concurrent chemoradiation has largely replaced radical surgery as curative treatment for localized anal cancer. Control rates are similar, and many patients can avoid permanent stoma.

Follow-up

After successful treatment of colorectal cancer, follow-up is aimed at the detection of recurrent disease (up to 50% of patients) and development of metachronous tumours (approximately 10% of patients). A total colonoscopy should be performed before surgery for detecting synchronous lesions elsewhere, and surveillance colonoscopy to detect recurrent polyps after surgery within 2–3 months, and thereafter at intervals of 3–5 years until about 75 years of age, depending on patient comorbidity. Ultrasound

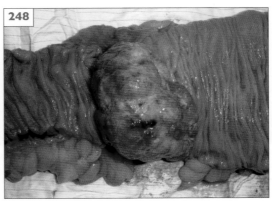

248 Operative specimen of carcinoma colon.

to detect asymptomatic metastases in the liver is sensible in the first 2 years following resection of the primary tumour. The roles of periodic chest radiograph, abdominal CT, or serum CEA levels to detect asymptomatic metastatic disease are uncertain.

Prevention
To prevent colon cancer, a number of different strategies can be adopted.

Low-risk groups
Routine screening of the middle-aged population can define the presence of polyps, or early cancers, after faecal occult blood screening or routine endoscopy (flexible sigmoidoscopy, rigid sigmoidoscopy, and full colonoscopy have all been advocated). Such approaches are expensive, but early detection and removal of adenomatous colonic polyps is the most effective means of improving prognosis.

High-risk groups
Screening groups with higher risk of colorectal cancer (previous polyps, family history of cancer at an early age or in more than one relative) leads to a higher yield of malignant or premalignant disease. Some dietary habits (high calcium intake, high fibre, less red meat) may be preventative and are under assessment, as is continuous low-dose acetylsalicylic acid orally.

Familial colorectal cancer syndromes

The majority (70–80%) of colorectal cancer occurs sporadically, and is related to age, diet, and environmental factors. In such patients, the genetic component is weak. In approximately 15–20% of colorectal cancer cases, there is a familial tendency, with a history of two family members affected by colorectal cancer, but no defined cancer syndrome. These conditions are assumed to be polygenetic, with low penetrance (often skipping a generation); no specific genes have been identified yet. Hereditary colorectal cancer syndromes contribute about 5% of colorectal cancers, but are monogenic disorders with high penetrance and early onset of cancer. They include HNPCC and a series of polyposis syndromes. The genes for some of these disorders have been defined; if identified in a proband, they can be used to assess risk in other family members.

Hereditary nonpolyposis colorectal cancer – HNPCC

HNPCC involves autosomal dominant genetic disorders, caused by mutations in one of the DNA mismatch repair genes. Affected kindreds can be identified empirically, or by analysis of characterization of the gene mutation. Unlike sporadic colorectal cancer, HNPCC tends to develop more proximal colonic lesions, presenting at a younger age. Different national bodies offer different recommendations. In the UK, the recommendations are colonoscopic surveillance biennially, starting 5 years before the age of the index case, or at 25 years old (whichever is the earlier). For those families in which gastric cancer occurs, upper gastrointestinal surveillance should start 5 years before the age of the index case, or at 50 years old (whichever is the earlier). Surveillance should be continued until 75 years old, or until the putative gene in this family has been excluded. Screening for extracolonic disease (especially endometrial) also needs to be considered.

Polyposis syndromes – mainly inherited

FAMILIAL ADENOMATOUS POLYPOSIS

FAP (**249–253**) syndromes are transmitted in an autosomal dominant fashion, with high penetrance. The adenomatous polyposis coli (*APC*) gene is located on chromosome 5, and a large number of mutations have been described. Colon polyps begin to appear in the early teens, and gastrointestinal symptoms in the third or fourth decades of life. The colon is studded with hundreds or thousands of polyps, and colon carcinoma develops by the age of 40 years in virtually all patients. Upper gastrointestinal polyps are common (stomach, mostly hyperplastic polyps (see **87, 88**); duodenum, 80% adenomatous polyps with periampullary carcinoma in 10%). Eye lesions caused by congenital hypertrophy of the retinal pigment epithelium (CHRPE) (**251**) are found in 80% of patients.

There are attenuated forms of FAP, with fewer polyps and a later cancer presentation.

Gardner syndrome

A subtype of familial polyposis, the Gardner syndrome is characterized by benign extra-intestinal growths, osteomas (mandibular), soft tissue tumours (lipomas, sebaceous cysts, fibrosarcomas), supernumerary teeth (**252**) desmoid tumours (**253**), and mesenteric fibromatosis.

Management

Colectomy is indicated when polyps appear in individuals with FAP, usually between the ages of 16 years and 20 years. If the rectum is retained following surgery, this will require ongoing surveillance. Until recently, flexible sigmoidoscopy on an annual basis was deemed necessary in all first-degree relatives between the ages of 12 years and 40 years, and every 3 years subsequently. Although, in the future, genetic analysis for *APC* mutations may allow relatives to be 'cleared' from risk, currently the *APC* mutation cannot be identified in every FAP family. Endoscopic surveillance for gastric and duodenal polyps is recommended every 2–3 years when colonic polyps develop. Additional interventions, depending upon complications, may be required by patients with Gardner syndrome.

PEUTZ–JEGHER'S SYNDROME

Peutz–Jegher's syndrome (**254**) is transmitted as autosomal dominant, with variable penetrance. Some kindreds have a mutation of a serine threonine kinase STK-11 (LKB1). Hamartomatous polyps may extend from the stomach to the rectum. Melanotic spots are found on the lips, buccal mucosa, and skin. Polyps are relatively sparse and exhibit a branching glandular pattern with smooth muscle proliferation. Different national bodies offer different recommendations. In the UK, the recommendations suggest 3-yearly colonoscopic surveillance from the age of 18 years.

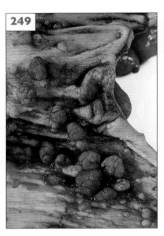

249 Resection specimen of the colon showing multiple polyps and familial polyposis.

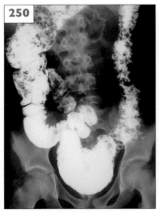

250 Familial polyposis on single-contrast barium enema. Note the numerous rounded polypoid filling defects, particularly in the ascending colon.

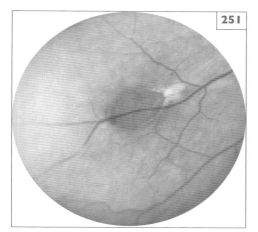

251 Fundoscopy showing CHRPE.

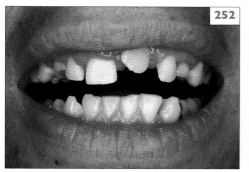

252 Abnormal dentition in familial polyposis coli.

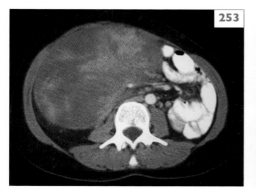

253 Some patients with familial polyposis coli have desmoid tumours. This is an intra-abdominal desmoid (not a liver!).

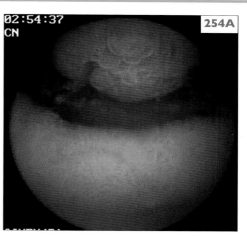

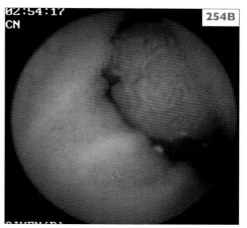

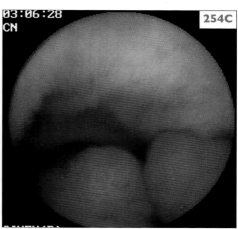

254 Three wireless capsule endoscopy pictures showing the small-intestinal polyps of Peutz–Jegher's syndrome.

Presentations are of gastrointestinal bleeding, colicky abdominal pain, and intussusception. Rare associations include small-intestinal and pancreatic malignancy, ovarian stromal tumours, and gallbladder, ureteric, or nasal polyps.

TURCOT'S SYNDROME

This is an autosomal recessive or dominant disorder, with abnormalities in the APC gene plus the nucleotide mismatch repair gene. The disorder is rare. Characteristic features are a lower number of colonic polyps than classical FAP, and the presence of CNS tumours, such as medulloblastoma, glioblastoma, and ependymoma.

JUVENILE POLYPOSIS

This is usually transmitted as an autosomal dominant disorder, but occasionally in a sporadic manner. Polyps number 25–40, and may be either restricted to the colon or involve the entire gastrointestinal tract. Rectal bleeding, iron-deficiency anaemia, abdominal pain, or intussusception may be presenting features in early childhood or adolescence. Congenital malformations may be noted, including pulmonary arteriovenous malformations and hereditary haemorrhagic telangiectasia (HHT). Juvenile polyposis syndromes are genetically heterogeneous and overlap with other hamartomatous syndromes; mutations in *SMAD4* and *BMP1RA* account for some kindreds. Approximately 10% of those affected develop gastrointestinal cancer; colonoscopic surveillance every 1–2 years from the age of 15–18 years, together with upper gastrointestinal endoscopic surveillance from the age of 25 years, has been recommended. Subtotal colectomy is often necessary.

CRONKHITE–CANADA SYNDROME

This is a nonfamilial disorder affecting adults. Polyps are commonly distributed in the stomach and colon. Other features are alopecia, fingernail dystrophy, and cutaneous hyperpigmentation. Watery diarrhoea, anorexia, abdominal pain, cachexia, and protein-losing enteropathy are manifestations, with gastrointestinal cancers in 14% of patients.

COWDEN'S SYNDROME

This is an autosomal dominant disorder with multiple hamartomas, facial tricholemmomas, oral papillomas (**255**), keratoses of the hands and feet, and nondysplastic colonic polyps without increase in colon cancer but with malignancy in other organs, e.g. thyroid and breast. Mutation in the tumour suppressor gene *PTEN* is present in the majority of patients.

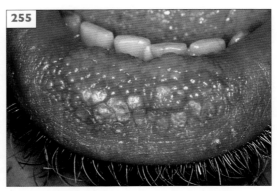

255 A patient with Cowden's syndrome (papillomata).

Ulcerative colitis

Definition

This is a chronic inflammatory condition of unknown aetiology, affecting a portion of or the entire colon (**256–258**). Ulcerative colitis may on occasion be indistinguishable from Crohn's colitis.

Epidemiology and aetiology

Although genetic and immunological mechanisms play important roles, the precise aetiology remains unknown. The disease afflicts all age groups, with a bimodal distribution, peaking between the second and third decades (the majority) or sixth and eighth decades. Ulcerative colitis is most common in northern Europe and America, as well as in European emigrants elsewhere. Ashkenazi Jews originating in Europe, compared with Sephardim, are more often affected. Ulcerative colitis is rare in Central or South America, Africa, the Middle East and Asia. However, no ethnic group is immune and the incidence of ulcerative colitis increases in black, Hispanic or Asian immigrants domiciled in high-incidence areas. Inflammatory bowel disease may show clustering in families. Offspring of two parents with the disease have a significant (40–50%) chance of acquiring inflammatory bowel disease. No specific genetic mode of transmission has been identified, although several genetic susceptibility loci have been suggested. Cigarette smoking may protect against ulcerative colitis; indeed, colitis may develop for the first time upon cessation of smoking. Environmental factors, including colonic bacteria, are most likely involved in inflammatory bowel disease.

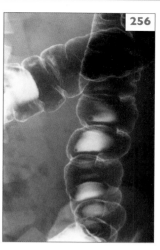

256 Barium enema showing diffuse ulcerative colitis, with multiple ulcers and a shaggy irregular mucosa.

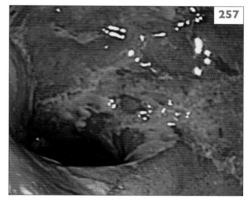

257 Endoscopic appearance of acute ulcerative colitis.

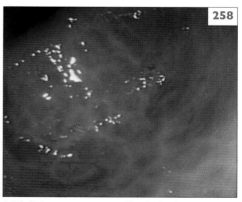

258 Colonoscopy view of healed colitis; sometimes this reticulated scarring is seen.

Pathophysiology

Multiple proinflammatory processes occur in the mucosa of ulcerative colitis, including T-cell proliferation, antibody production, and expression of inflammatory mediators, such as leukotrienes, platelet-activating factor, histamine, kinins, chemotactic substances, and neuropeptides. The end result is mucosal inflammation, exudation of an inflammatory infiltrate containing neutrophils, epithelial necrosis, and ulceration. The inflammatory infiltrate is most pronounced in the lamina propria and epithelium, without being transmural. Accumulation of the inflammatory exudate between adjacent crypts generates 'crypt abscesses', and goblet cells are depleted of mucus (**259, 260**). Repeated injury and repair ultimately lead to fibrosis (**258**) and thinning of the colonic wall, loss of haustrations (lead pipe appearance), and occasional development of strictures. Areas of hyperplastic mucosa in the setting of ongoing inflammation appear as 'pseudopolyps' at endoscopy (**261**). Mucosal epithelial cells may demonstrate nuclear atypia (dysplastic change), with an increased risk for colon carcinoma (**262, 263**).

Left-sided colitis, involving the rectum and sigmoid colon, is most frequent (25–50%); the rectum alone may be involved (25%), or inflammation may extend proximal to the splenic flexure and produce pancolitis (25–30%).

Occasionally, proctitis may accompany patches of colitis in the caecum or right colon. The inflamed segments of the colon are diffusely involved, in contrast to discontinuous involvement and skip areas in Crohn's colitis. The ileum is not affected in ulcerative colitis, although inflammatory exudate may flow into the ileum producing so-called 'backwash ileitis'.

Clinical history

The onset of an attack is usually insidious, depending upon disease extent and severity. Proctitis manifests with tenesmus and semi-solid stools containing blood, mucus, and pus. Diarrhoea, abdominal pain, cramping, or distension, and localized tenderness are additional features of more extensive disease. Systemic symptoms may occur, such as fever, malaise, nausea, vomiting, night sweats, and arthralgias. Coexisting constipation or irritable colon syndrome may mask manifestations of ulcerative colitis. Severe colitis is characterized

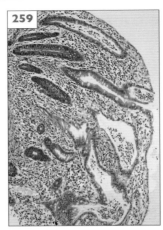

259 Biopsy specimen of acute ulcerative colitis showing diffuse inflammatory infiltrate, loss of surface epithelium, loss of mucin, and crypt abscesses (neutrophils in the gland spaces).

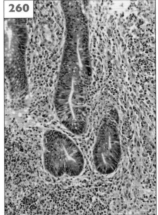

260 Histological section of active ulcerative colitis. Note the distorted gland architecture and branching glands, indicating that regeneration has taken place.

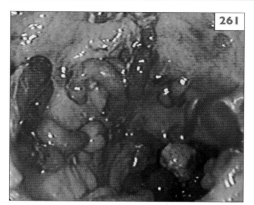

261 Endoscopic appearance of pseudopolyp (regenerative epithelium).

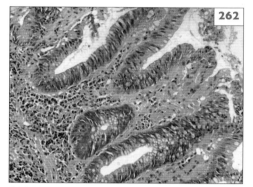

262 Histological sections of ulcerative colitis showing dysplasia. The nuclei at the base of the epithelial cells are larger and the nuclear layer is more than one layer thick.

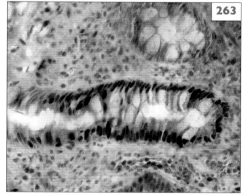

263 Strong p53 nuclear immunostaining in the crypts of dysplastic ulcerative colitis mucosa.

by increased bowel frequency, blood in stools, fever, tachycardia, anaemia, rising ESR, marked abdominal tenderness, decreased bowel sounds and colonic dilatation. Clinical features of severe disease (*Table 3*) indicate that a patient should be admitted to hospital for treatment, including notably the use of intravenous steroids.

Physical examination

There may be evidence of weight loss, eye abnormalities such as uveitis, skin rashes, pyoderma gangrenosum, arthritis, finger clubbing, and localized or diffuse abdominal tenderness with or without abdominal distension.

Laboratory and special examinations

With increasing severity and length of relapses, there may be peripheral leukocytosis, anaemia of chronic disease or of iron deficiency, thrombocythaemia, fluid and electrolyte imbalances (particularly hypokalaemia), hypoalbuminaemia secondary to PLE, evidence of systemic inflammation (raised ESR, acute phase response proteins), and elevated serum alkaline phosphatase, aminotransferases or gamma-glutamyltransferase (GGT) in case of coexisting hepatitis or cholangitis.

Table 3 Clinical characteristics of severe colitis

Diarrhoea	Six times daily
Macroscopic blood	+++
Temperature	>38°C
Pulse	>100/min
ESR	>30 mm/h
Hb	<11 g/dl

Imaging

Plain abdominal radiographs may show thickened and oedematous bowel mucosa (**264**), or complications such as toxic megacolon (transverse colon >6 cm) or colonic perforation (free air under the diaphragm). A barium enema may demonstrate mucosal ulceration or irregularity, and colonic shortening with loss of haustral pattern in chronic disease (**265**) Barium enema is ill-advised in acute colitis, as it may precipitate toxic megacolon (see below). CT scanning is sometimes appropriate.

Endoscopy

Sigmoidoscopy and rectal biopsy are extremely helpful for demonstrating characteristic endoscopic and histological features. The mucosa is diffusely erythematous and friable, with punctate ulcerations and mucopus. Skip lesions (intervening normal mucosa within an area of inflammation) are not a feature. Pseudopolyps, stricture, or cancer may be encountered. A colonoscopy may be necessary for defining the extent of the disease. Colonic evaluation is appropriate in all except the most seriously ill patients, who are at risk of toxic megacolon.

Nuclear medicine

White cell scans using indium 111- or ^{99m}Tc-labelled autologous leukocytes facilitate noninvasive localization of colonic inflammation (**266**). A timed stool collection and measurement of radioactivity in the stool can provide a quantitative assessment of inflammation.

Complications

Toxic megacolon

This is colonic dilatation, with impaired viability of the colonic wall due to secondary bacterial infection, hypoperfusion, and stasis; it is a complication of severe colitis. Precipitating factors include hypokalaemia, anticholinergic or narcotic drugs, barium enema, or air instillation during endoscopy. Early warning signs in plain X-ray are loss of bowel tone, with accumulation of gas over long segments of the colon, before dilatation occurs. The syndrome of toxic megacolon develops with increased abdominal pain or distension, rebound tenderness, hypovolaemia, leukocytosis, or septic shock. Colonic perforation may be a late feature.

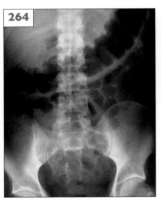

264 Plain X-ray – there is oedematous bowel wall and no gas in the descending colon.

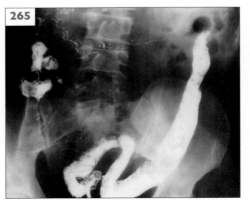

265 Single-contrast barium enema showing a tubular featureless left colon of a patient with chronic inflammatory bowel disease.

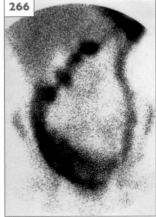

266 White cell scan showing diffuse inflammation throughout the transverse, descending colon and the rectum in active pancolitis.

Colon carcinoma

Colon carcinoma (**267**) may develop in the setting of long-standing disease (usually >10 years). Mucosal dysplasia in the absence of chronic inflammatory changes is sinister and constitutes a precancerous lesion requiring resection.

Extraintestinal complications

These may be grouped as follows:

- Nutritional and metabolic: PLE, weight loss, and growth retardation (especially in the young).
- Haematological: iron-deficiency anaemia, leukocytosis, and thrombocytosis.
- Cutaneous: stomatitis with aphthous ulcers, erythema nodosum, and pyoderma gangrenosum (indolent ulcer on extremities with vaso-occlusive features, hyperpigmentation, undermined edges, and superinfection of the exudate) (**268**).
- Musculoskeletal: HLA-B27-associated arthropathies, such as ankylosing spondylitis (**269, 270**) or sacroiliitis, arthritis involving peripheral large joints, and osteoporosis.
- Hepatic: fatty liver, sclerosing cholangitis, cholangiocarcinoma.
- Renal: nephrolithiasis.
- Ocular: conjunctivitis, episcleritis, iritis, uveitis.
- Obstetric: reduced fertility, increased foetal loss.

With increasing severity and length of relapses, there may be peripheral leukocytosis and anaemia of chronic disease.

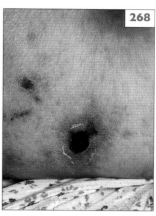

268 Pyoderma gangrenosum, a systemic complication of inflammatory bowel disease.

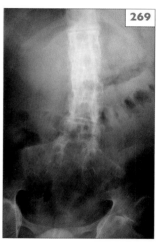

269 Spondylitis; there is sclerosis and obliteration of the normal sacroiliac joint.

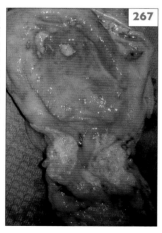

267 Operative specimen of long-standing ulcerative colitis and a complicating colon carcinoma.

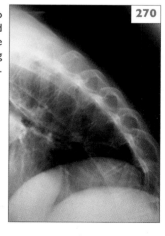

270 'Bamboo spine' – rigid ankylosed spine of ankylosing spondylitis.

Differential diagnosis

Differentiate from Crohn's disease (*Table 4*), infectious proctitis, colitis due to viral (e.g. CMV), bacterial, fungal, or parasitic aetiologies, diverticulitis, radiation colitis, vasculitis, and drug- or toxin-induced enterocolitis.

Prognosis

The course is highly variable, ranging from a single symptomatic episode to recurrent exacerbations or unremitting inflammation and multiple intercurrent complications. Prognosis is determined by the extent and severity of bowel disease, coexisting medical disorders, and response to therapies. Toxic megacolon or perforation result in mortality rates of 20–30%. In the elderly, inflammatory bowel disease is not more severe, but outcomes may be worse due to coexisting cardiac, pulmonary, or other ailments.

Management

In remission

Maintain remission by oral 5-ASA. Sulfasalazine (sulphapyridine plus 5-ASA) is split by bacteria in the colon to release 5-ASA, but is poorly tolerated in some patients, causing nausea, rashes, male infertility, and (rarely) agranulocytosis. Alternative 5-ASA preparations (mesalazine, olsalazine, and balsalazide) deliver the drug to the colon without sulphapyridine; they confer a small risk of interstitial nephritis.

Acute attacks

There is some beneficial effect from oral 5-ASA, but additional treatment is generally needed:

- Distal disease: requires suppositories, foam, or aqueous enemas of 5-ASA or prednisolone (or other steroid).
- Extensive or severe disease: requires systemic steroids, given orally or intravenously.
- Severe colitis (*Table 3*) is a medical emergency needing admission, intravenous fluids, high-dose parenteral steroids, and sometimes ciclosporin.

Additional immunosuppressive agents, such as 6-mercaptopurine (6-MP) or azathioprine are useful for corticosteroid-dependent or corticosteroid-resistant colitis. Infliximab has also proved to have a role.

Surgery

This is necessary in the acute setting for unremitting acute colitis, toxic megacolon, and colonic perforation (**271**). Elective surgery is appropriate for definite dysplasia or cancer (**246**). The classical surgical procedure of proctocolectomy and ileostomy is now less

Table 4 Differences between Crohn's disease and ulcerative colitis

	Ulcerative colitis	Crohn's disease
History of smoking	+/–	++
Perianal disease	–	+++
Ileal involvement	–	++
Strictures	+/–	++
Cured by colectomy	+++	–
Endoscopy		
Rectal disease	+++	+
Diffuse and continuous disease	+++	+
Aphthous ulcers	–	+++
Cobblestoning	–	++
Pathology		
Transmural disease	–	+++
Lymphoid aggregates	–	+++
Granulomas	–	++
Fistula	–	+++

commonly performed, and colectomy can be done via a laparoscopic approach. Sphincter-saving procedures providing continence have gained better patient acceptance. The ileoanal pouch procedure provides for normal rectal passage of stool, although faecal frequency and some faecal seepage are common.

Colonic surveillance by colonoscopy

The role for colonoscopic surveillance must be discussed with each patient. Different national bodies offer different recommendations. In the UK, the recommendation is a colonoscopy 8–10 years after diagnosis to define the macroscopic extent of disease. In patients with pancolitis, surveillance colonoscopy should be every 3 years in the second decade of disease, every 2 years in the third decade, and yearly by the fourth decade. For patients with left-sided disease, in whom the cancer risk is lower, surveillance is suggested only after 15–20 years of disease. Patients with PSC (especially if they undergo liver transplantation) are at particular risk of colonic cancer and require more frequent colonoscopy.

Surveillance colonoscopy should be undertaken during quiescence as regenerative atypia can be misinterpreted as dysplasia. Dysplasia should be confirmed by two pathologists, as there is a significant rate of cancer in explants for this indication. Dysplasia-associated lesions of mass (DALM) and flat lesions with high-grade dysplasia are definite indications for colectomy. The management of low-grade dysplasia is less clear cut, with most authorities recommending colectomy as opposed to more intensive surveillance.

Pregnancy tends to exacerbate ulcerative colitis, although the risks have been overemphasized. It is safe to continue sulfasalazine in pregnancy, and colitis is usually controlled with corticosteroids.

Proctitis

In proctitis, inflammation similar to that seen in ulcerative colitis may be limited to the lower few centimetres of the rectum. This form probably constitutes about half the cases seen in ambulatory populations. There is often a sharp demarcation between normal and abnormal mucosa. This is now generally thought to be a subtype of ulcerative colitis; over 10 years, 10–30% of patients experience proximal extension of the inflammation.

Treatment is as for ulcerative colitis, but with a greater dependence on local therapies (5-ASA suppositories, local steroids).

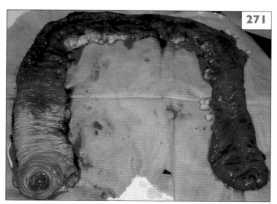

271 Colonic resection for acute fulminant colitis – the colon is continuously inflamed proximally from the rectum.

Microscopic colitis

Definition
Microscopic colitis is defined as chronic watery diarrhoea with normal colonic mucosa at endoscopy or radiology, but with chronic mucosal inflammation evident on histology.

Epidemiology and aetiology
The usual age of onset is 60–65 years, and females are much more frequently affected. There may be associated systemic disorders, such as arthritis, autoimmune disease, or thyroid disorders. The precise aetiology of collagenous colitis or variants is unknown. Some features of colonic injury resemble those produced by NSAIDs or other drugs – including proton pump inhibitors.

Pathophysiology
Variants of microscopic colitis include lymphocytic colitis and collagenous colitis. The characteristic feature of collagenous colitis is a thickened subepithelial collagen band, whereas in lymphocytic colitis there is infiltration of the mucosa by lymphocytic infiltrates (272–274). Some patients have mixed features. In addition, some patients have similar inflammatory changes in the small bowel, along with subtotal villous atrophy that resembles coeliac disease and suggests shared pathogenetic mechanisms. However, unlike coeliac disease, the colonic inflammation does not respond to a gluten-restricted diet. Also, there is no association between collagenous colitis and HLA-B8/DR3, which are highly prevalent in coeliac disease. Colonic histology is diagnostic. The crypt architecture is preserved, with increased intraepithelial lymphocytes, mildly decreased goblet cells, and only rare neutrophils. Deposition of a layer of type IV collagen in the subepithelial region of the colonic mucosa is most characteristic of collagenous colitis. The band of collagen may be as thick as 100 μm, with deposition most frequent in the caecum or transverse colon (>80% of cases) and least in the rectum (<30%). Unlike ulcerative colitis, crypt abscesses are not seen.

Clinical history
Patients report chronic, watery diarrhoea without blood for months or years. Faecal incontinence, nocturnal stools, crampy abdominal pain, nausea, and weight loss may be prominent.

Physical examination
There are no specific changes.

Laboratory and special examinations
Typically, expect mild anaemia, hypoalbuminaemia, and elevated ESR. Steatorrhoea is rare. Full colonoscopy is indicated, as the distribution of the disease can be patchy and can be overlooked if only rectosigmoid biopsies are taken. Multiple colonic biopsies are taken and provide the diagnosis.

Differential diagnosis
Differentiate from ulcerative colitis, Crohn's disease, infectious colitis, giardiasis, and coeliac disease. The normal endoscopic findings macroscopically are an important diagnostic feature.

Prognosis
No cures are available. The course is variable and the disease usually remains indolent.

Management
Treatment is empiric. Some patients may benefit from cessation of NSAIDs or other causative drugs. Loperamide or other antidiarrhoeals are used. Sulfasalazine, 5-ASA, and budesonide or corticosteroids may help in controlling symptoms, but do not reverse collagen deposition.

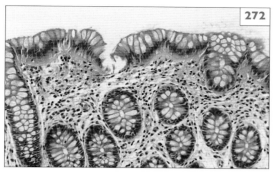

272 Normal colonic histology.

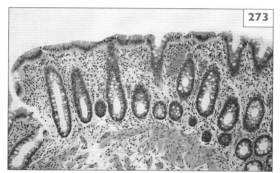

273 Histopathological appearances of the colon in collagenous colitis. Note the thick pink area behind the mucosal epithelial layer (collagen). Compare with **272**.

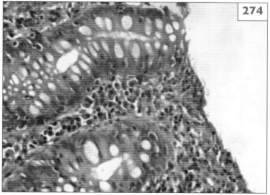

274 Excessive intraepithelial lymphocytes without crypt distortion in lymphocytic colitis.

Radiation colitis

Definition
Radiation colitis is defined as characteristic colonic injury after exposure to ionizing radiation, usually manifesting acutely during radiotherapy, and also months or years later in an insidious form. (See Chapter 5 for a discussion of radiation enteritis.)

Epidemiology and aetiology
Radiation damage to the bowel usually occurs after exposure to a cumulative dose of 50 Gy (5,000 rads). Cells entering DNA synthesis or mitosis are particularly sensitive to radiation injury. External radiation to pelvic organs inevitably exposes portions of the bowel to injury. Brachytherapy (internal radiation with implanted sources) is a safer alternative, as the radiation beam is attenuated. The colon is relatively radioresistant, but is most affected by radiation due to the relative immobility of the rectosigmoid region and difficulty in protecting the area while irradiating other organs, especially the prostate.

Pathophysiology
The earliest changes involve microscopic damage to the epithelial cells and vascular endothelial cells, marked submucosal oedema secondary to increased vascular permeability, and superficial ulcerations. In persistent radiation damage, ulceration is extended, vascular endothelium proliferates with telangiectasia, and granulation tissue appears, along with atypical fibroblasts and collagen deposition. Endothelial inflammation and intimal proliferation lead to obliterative arteriopathy. Eventually, the bowel wall atrophies, fibrosis develops, and complicating strictures, fistula, or leaks occur. Proctosigmoiditis is most common (75%).

Clinical history
Acute radiation proctosigmoiditis presents with diarrhoea, tenesmus, and rarely bleeding, and usually resolves within 2–6 months.

Chronic colitis presents with rectal pain, diarrhoea, and bleeding, usually within 2 years of irradiation, but occasionally after decades.

Physical examination
There are no specific abnormalities.

Laboratory and special examinations
Digital rectal examination may be painful. Endoscopy demonstrates pale mucosa, friability, and telangiectasia. Discrete ulceration is rare (275, 276). Endoscopic biopsies usually do not display characteristic features of radiation injury, as these usually involve deeper tissues (277). Barium or gastrograffin enemas may be helpful in demonstrating strictures, fistulae, or leaks.

Differential diagnosis
Differentiate from other colitides, including infectious and ulcerative colitis.

Prognosis
The spontaneous rates of remission are lower in the presence of significant bleeding or anaemia requiring blood transfusion. Surgery is required in approximately 50% of cases, but may be dangerous. Recurrent disease is frequent after surgery, and urinary complications are particularly troublesome.

Management
Anti-inflammatory agents, such as sulfasalazine, corticosteroids, or sucralfate enemas are tried but usually do not help. Dilatation of strictures may be required. Surgery (resection and reanastomosis or anteroposterior resection) may be required, but is often complicated by leaks or sepsis. Mortality rates of up to 60% have been reported.

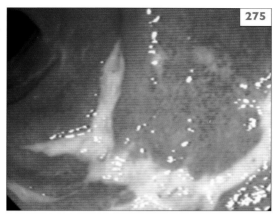

275 Acute radiation proctitis following radiotherapy for prostatic cancer.

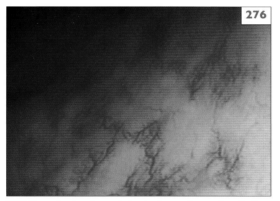

276 Rectal telangiectasia in the later phase of radiation proctitis.

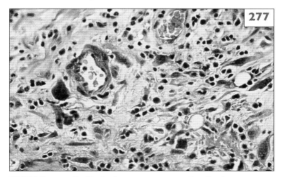

277 Histopathological appearances of radiation enteritis. There are large bizarre fibroblasts showing effects of radiation.

Infectious colitis and proctocolitis

Definition

Infection with bacteria, such as *Shigella, Campylobacter*, and enteroinvasive or enterohaemorrhagic *Escherichia coli*, produces an acute colitis. *Clostridium difficile* infection causes pseudomembranous or antibiotic-associated colitis. Acute infectious proctitis may be due to *Chlamydia trachomatis, Neisseria gonorrhoeae, Treponema pallidum*, amoebiasis, or HSV type 1.

SHIGELLOSIS

This causes bacillary dysentery due to Shiga exotoxins. Aerobic Gram-negative bacilli fall into four major serotypes: *S. dysenteriae, S. boydii, S. flexneri*, and *S. sonnei*. Transmission is by the oro-faecal route. Shigellosis is prevalent worldwide, with a high attack rate after exposure (60%). The condition is endemic in India, South East Asia, and Mexico. Young children, travellers, and institutional residents are most susceptible. Infection is less frequent in developed countries, although approximately 300,000 cases occur annually in the United States. The incubation period is 1–3 days. Typically, the illness is short lived and resolves spontaneously. However, a subacute waxing and waning course, lasting 2–3 weeks, may be observed. Complications may occur, such as Reiter's syndrome (arthritis, nonspecific urethritis, and conjunctivitis), as well as ankylosing spondylitis (in HLA-B27 carriers) and, rarely, haemolytic uraemic syndrome (acute haemolytic anaemia, renal failure, and disseminated intravascular coagulation).

CAMPYLOBACTER JEJUNI

This is an important cause of bacterial colitis (approximately 20% of cases). The Gram-negative, motile bacteria are transmitted through the oro-faecal route via contaminated poultry, milk, eggs, or exposure to sick pets. *C. jejuni* is now a leading cause of food-related gastroenteritis. Children younger than 5 years old are most frequently affected. The incubation period is 1–6 days, with a prodrome associated with influenza-like symptoms, high fevers, aches, and confusion. The infection is usually a short-lived gastroenteritis, but may range from asymptomatic individuals to severe and life-threatening disease with toxic megacolon, pseudomembranous colitis, exacerbation of inflammatory bowel disease, and Reiter's syndrome. Abdominal pain may be severe. A relapsing course with rectal bleeding may be seen, although stool cultures tend to be negative after 5 weeks in 90% of patients. A postinfective irritable bowel syndrome is more frequent in females with a long index illness. Complications, including Guillain–Barré syndrome, haemolytic uraemic syndrome, reactive arthritides (especially in those with HLA-B27), and acute cholecystitis, are all reported rarely.

ESCHERICHIA COLI

This infection (with Gram-negative bacilli) is due either to the enteroinvasive *E. coli* (15% of cases) producing 'traveller's diarrhoea', or to the enterohaemorrhagic *E. coli* (O157:H7) strain. Traveller's diarrhoea, which results from mucosal damage by the invasive bacteria, is usually mild, lasts for 1–3 days, and may be prevented by antibiotics, such as doxycycline. The O157:H7 strain causes disease by releasing exotoxins. Strain O157:H7, which may be transmitted by uncooked ground beef (e.g. hamburgers), dairy products, drinking water, or close contact with farm animals causes profuse diarrhoea accompanied by blood after 12–24 hours. Feared complications of haemolytic uraemic syndrome and thrombotic thrombocytopenic purpura may cause fatalities. Several stool cultures may be needed for diagnosis.

CLOSTRIDIUM DIFFICILE

These Gram-positive bacilli cause disease when the normal bowel flora is altered, such as by antibiotics (particularly penicillin), cancer chemotherapy, or another pathogen. The bacteria produce heat-labile exotoxins – toxin A (250 kDa mass) and toxin B (309 kDa mass) – the latter being approximately 100 times more potent. The toxins are detectable by bio- or immunoassays, both of which are more convenient than culture of the fastidious organism. Occasionally, bacterial toxins may be detected in nonpathogenic settings. There have been recent reports of more virulent strains of *C. difficile* strains with a mutant *txcD* gene, producing far more toxin. *C. difficile* infection often complicates inflammatory bowel disease and is responsible for 5–25% of the exacerbations. The histological lesions of pseudomembranous colitis (*C. difficile* infection) are highly characteristic, with prominent outpouring, from microulcerated areas in the mucosa, of fibrinous exudate containing copious neutrophils (summit or volcano lesion) (**278**). Clinical manifestations of *C. difficile* infection may range from asymptomatic states, to antibiotic-associated watery diarrhoea and pseudomembranous colitis (**279**).

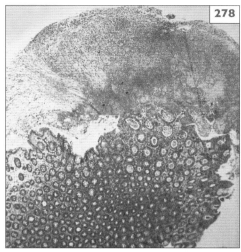

278 Histopathological appearances of pseudomembranous colitis (so-called 'volcano lesion'), the pseudomembrane consisting of polymorphonuclear leukocytes.

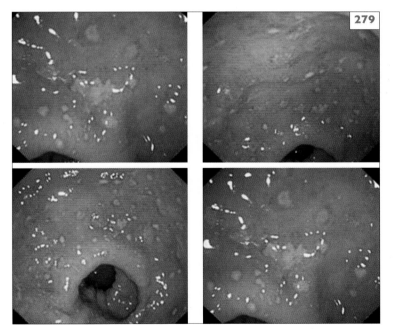

279 Endoscopic appearances of yellow pseudomembranes in *Clostridium difficile* infection (pseudomembranous colitis).

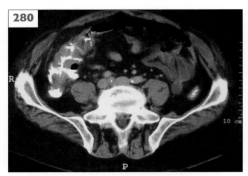

280 Fulminant colitis caused by *Clostridium difficile*. There is oedema and wall thickening in the ascending colon.

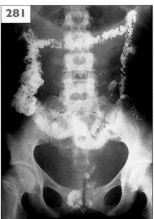

281 Diffuse mucosal thickening and irregularity throughout the colon, in this case showing the presence of tuberculous colitis. The terminal small intestine is also abnormal, due to lymphangiectasia secondary to tuberculosis.

When fulminant, *C. difficile* infection may be life-threatening with marked debilitation, constitutional symptoms, grossly raised inflammatory indices, leukocytosis, and toxic megacolon, colonic perforation, or paralytic ileus (**280**).

Treatment consists of stopping the precipitating antibiotics when this is feasible, with oral metronidazole for 10 days as the first-line therapy. Oral vancomycin, although more expensive, may show slightly greater efficacy (90–95%) than oral or intravenous metronidazole (85–90%). Relapses of *C. difficile* infection are common (around 30%) and may require repeat courses of the same antibiotic or a switch to another. If the relapse is after initial treatment with metronidazole, it is generally accepted that vancomycin should be substituted. Alternative agents for treating *C. difficile* infection are rifampicin, fusidin, bacitracin and teicoplanin. There are anecdotal reports of immunoglobulin infusions for refractory infection. Colectomy is reserved for fulminant cases.

TUBERCULOSIS

Tuberculosis may affect the colon, with *Mycobacterium tuberculosis* of bovine or human strain. The clinical features are those of diarrhoea, pain, and bleeding, and have been discussed in Chapter 5. Colonic tuberculosis is diagnosed by a colonoscopy and biopsy with culture, and may be suspected from barium enema findings (**179, 180, 281, 282**).

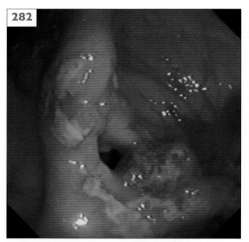

282 Discrete ulceration in the ascending colon at colonoscopy – in this case due to tuberculosis.

ACUTE INFECTIOUS PROCTITIS

This condition is usually encountered in the setting of venereal infection in the homosexual or the immunocompromised. Herpetic proctitis is the usual form in homosexuals. The general manifestations of proctitis may accompany more typical features of infection, e.g. inguinal lymphadenopathy in the setting of lymphogranuloma venereum (*Chlamydia trachomatis*), anal canal chancre (syphilis), or anal warts (human papilloma virus, HPV), although the disease may be localized to the rectum alone, such as in gonorrhoeal proctitis or amoebiasis. Simultaneous evaluation of the genital organs of the patient, and of the contacts (when feasible), is indicated.

Pathophysiology

The mechanisms common to most infectious colitides involve adhesion of microbes to the bowel wall and epithelial damage, due either to the release of exotoxins or to direct cytotoxicity. In comparison with chronic ulcerative colitis, mucin depletion in goblet cells is not as prominent, crypt abscesses are not seen, inflammatory changes tend not to extend to the lamina propria, and specific agents, such as viruses or parasites, may be identified.

Clinical history

The characteristic common features are tenesmus (incomplete sense of bowel evacuation), cramping lower abdominal pain, and small-volume diarrhoea with blood, mucus, and leukocytes in the stool. In proctitis, rectal pain is prominent and urinary symptoms, such as retention or poor stream, may develop. Fever and constitutional symptoms occur in severe disease. History of antibiotic ingestion in the preceding few weeks or even months (*C. difficile*), homosexual activity (venereal proctitis), or immunocompromised state (HSV type 1 proctitis, amoebiasis, etc.) may be elicited.

Physical examination

Patients should be examined for fever, tenderness in the left lower quadrant of the abdomen, painful rectal examination with blood, mucus, or pus, and possibly features of dehydration.

Laboratory and special examinations

Typically features are peripheral blood leukocytosis and mild anaemia. The presence of leukocytes in the stool markedly increases the possibility of a positive stool culture. Detection of *C. difficile* toxins in the stool is more convenient than bacterial culture. Sigmoidoscopy reveals erythema, friability, diffuse or typical mucosal ulceration, and exudates or pseudomembranes. Rectal biopsy is diagnostic when characteristic changes are found, e.g. pseudomembranous colitis or cytomegalovirus (**283, 284**), whereas

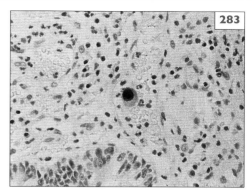

283 A large cell, staining positively for CMV antibodies, in a patient with CMV colitis.

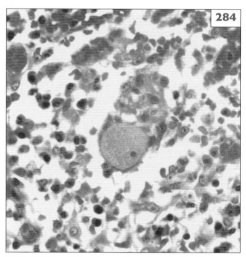

284 CMV colitis – here showing the 'owl's eye' inclusion body.

distinction between resolving bacterial and ulcerative colitis may occasionally be difficult. Radiological imaging is helpful only in advanced cases with toxic megacolon or other complications.

Differential diagnosis

Differentiate from inflammatory bowel disease, radiation- or drug-induced colitis, ischaemic colitis, and parasitic infestation.

Prognosis

Most patients with infectious colitis make a complete recovery. The onset of acute complications, such as haemolytic uraemic syndrome, is associated with poor prognosis, including fatalities. Complications, such as Reiter's syndrome, may be associated with a protracted symptomatic course. The most important consequences of infectious colitis involve the public health arena, in view of massive worldwide loss of productive activity.

Management

The mainstays are correction of dehydration, contact isolation, and prevention of infection in susceptible groups by public health measures. Specific therapeutic interventions are not necessary for all bacterial infections, as many resolve by themselves.

- Shigellosis may be treated by tetracyclines, ampicillin, or co-trimoxazole, as well as by quinolones (ciprofloxacin).
- *Campylobacter* infections are treated by erythromycin or ciprofloxacin.
- *E. coli* infections may be treated by co-trimoxazole, ampicillin, quinolones, and tetracycline.
- Lymphogranuloma venereum is treated by tetracycline, and gonorrhoea and syphilis by penicillin or cephalosporins.
- HSV type-1 is treated by aciclovir, and HPV by podophyllin or cryotherapy.
- CMV colitis can be treated with gancyclovir.

ACTINOMYCOSIS

Actinomyces is an uncommon, chronic, invasive Gram-positive filamentous organism. It is a commensal in the mouth and gut. In the gastrointestinal tract, it has a propensity for the craniofacial and ileocaecal regions. Here, it causes indolent suppurative granulomatous infection, with mass, local fistulae, sinus tracks that discharge 'sulphur granules', and perforation (**285**). Risk factors include recent abdominopelvic surgery (including gynaecological interventions such as intrauterine contraceptive device placement), neoplasia, and perforated viscus. Preoperative diagnosis is difficult, as actinomycosis mimics many other diseases. The presentation is usually nonspecific, and frequently the diagnosis is only made at laparotomy. The differential diagnosis is appendix mass, Crohn's disease, lymphoma, or carcinoma of the caecum. Pus microbiology can be diagnostic, and histology shows the *Actinomyces* surrounded by granuloma (**286**). Treatment is generally surgical, with prolonged antibiotic (penicillin). Mortality is rare.

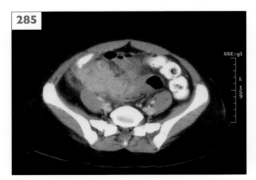

285 Actinomycosis presenting as a complex pelvic mass involving caecum, appendix, and right ovary.

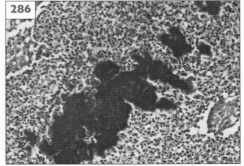

286 Actinomycosis histology of resected specimen.

Drug and chemical colitis

Definition
This condition is defined as colitis resulting from the direct action of soaps, water-soluble contrast media, hydrogen peroxide, acids, alkali, irritants, and laxatives or other agents. Mild injury not coming to medical attention may be far more frequent than severe injury. The public interest in 'colonic lavage' for improving health, and the incorporation of untested, exotic ingredients into cleansing enemas, may enhance the overall incidence of injury. Mild inflammation is common, but severe acute colitis, perforation, and cicatrization over 3–4 weeks may be seen.

MELANOSIS COLI
This refers to dark pigmentation of the colonic mucosa (**287**), with a reticulated appearance after exposure to anthraquinone laxatives (cascara, aloe, rhubarb, senna, frangula, etc.).

Epidemiology, aetiology, and pathophysiology
Melanosis is due to the deposition of brown, granular pigment consisting of melanin or lipofuscin within macrophages in the lamina propria. The number of macrophages increases between colonic crypts, with epithelial cells demonstrating apoptosis, as well as ultrastructural abnormalities of uncertain significance. Colonic melanosis requires an average of 9 months to develop, but may occur within 4 months, and resolves upon discontinuation of the incriminating agent. The overall prevalence is 0.25–24% of colonoscopies. Patients are typically above 40 years old, and female. The caecum and rectum are commonly affected, although the entire colon may be involved.

Clinical history
There are no specific symptoms.

Physical examination
There are no systemic or peripheral abnormalities.

Laboratory and special examinations
Endoscopy and biopsy are diagnostic. The colonic mucosa appears black or slate grey, with reticulated striations or spots reminiscent of alligator skin.

Differential diagnosis
There is no differential diagnosis.

Prognosis
This is a benign disorder. No increased cancer risk has been identified.

Management
Management is by removal of the incriminating agents.

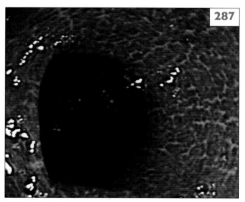

287 Colonic appearance in melanosis coli, reflecting laxative abuse.

Cathartic colon

Definition
Cathartic colon is defined as colonic sequelae of chronic laxative abuse.

Epidemiology and aetiology
The manifestations are related to persistent and excessive use of laxatives, such as anthraquinones. Patients may suffer from chronic constipation, preoccupation with bowel movements, psychological disturbances, or surreptitious drug use.

Pathophysiology
Persistent and excessive laxative intake damages the myenteric neural plexus with colonic dysmotility, as well as causing gross morphological alterations. The resulting rapid transit through the bowel may occasionally even manifest with impaired digestion (steatorrhoea or excess protein loss via the stool).

Clinical history
Typically, there is abdominal bloating or fullness, lower abdominal cramping pain, and diarrhoea or constipation. A history of excess laxative intake may not readily be elicited.

Physical examination
No specific examination is suggested.

Laboratory and special examinations
Patients should be examined for serum electrolyte abnormalities, such as hypo-kalaemia. A plain radiograph or barium enema demonstrates characteristic features, such as loss of haustra, foreshortening and conical shape of the caecum, and dilatation of the colon into a tubular shape (**288, 289**). Biopsies are usually normal. Melanosis coli may be an accompaniment, but not necessarily so. If laxative abuse is denied, chemical identification of laxatives in the urine may be helpful (**290**).

Differential diagnosis
Some morphological features may superficially resemble chronic ulcerative colitis, but the distinction is usually straightforward.

Prognosis
Resolution depends upon the ability to discontinue laxatives. Most changes resolve within a few months.

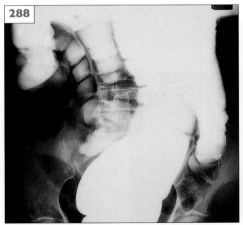

288 Megacolon, reflecting long-term laxative abuse.

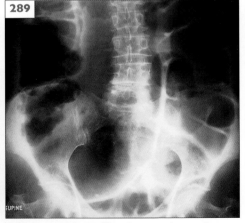

289 Gross colonic dilatation seen in a patient with megacolon due to laxatives. The maintenance of a normal haustral pattern differentiates this from toxic megacolon.

Management

Withdrawal of laxatives is most important. This usually requires bowel retraining, the use of bulking agents, and switching to osmotic laxatives or enemas. In refractory cases, recourse to drastic measures, such as total or subtotal colectomy may be required.

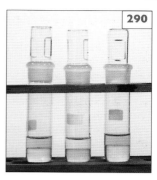

290 A positive anthracene test showing the presence of senna or one of its derivatives in a laxative-abusing patient.

Parasitic infestations of the colon

Definition

Amoebiasis, schistosomiasis, and Chagas' disease are most remarkable for involvement of the colon, as well as other organs. Pinworm or whipworm infestations are also frequent.

AMOEBIASIS

The causative agent is *Entamoeba histolytica*. A variety of saprophytic entamoebas, which only rarely cause disease, colonize humans, and a distinction must be made between these and the pathogenic *E. histolytica*.

Epidemiology and aetiology

After malaria and schistosomiasis, amoebiasis is the most prevalent parasitic disease in the world, accounting annually for more than 500 million cases, with colitis or liver abscess in approximately 50 million, and death in approximately 100,000 people. The greatest prevalence is in India, Africa and Central and South America. The groups at greatest risk are inhabitants of, or immigrants from, endemic areas, promiscuous male homosexuals, and the institutionalized.

Pathophysiology

The virulence depends upon the strain of *E. histolytica*, as well as on interactions with colonic bacteria and host-specific factors. After oro-faecal transmission of *E. histolytica* cysts, trophozoites arise through excystation and adhere to the colonic epithelium. The trophozoites release proteases and collagenases, as well as endotoxins, which result in mucosal inflammation, lysis, and a host immune response. The trophozoites may travel to the liver via the portal vein, producing an abscess. Exposure to *E. histolytica* generates long-lasting antibodies against surface antigens of the parasite, as well as T-lymphocyte responses that decrease recurrence of the disease; e.g. a second amoebic liver abscess is highly unusual (<3 cases/1,000).

Clinical history

Symptoms vary widely, depending upon the extent and nature of colonization. They include asymptomatic cyst carriers, which constitute reservoirs of infection. Manifestations include diarrhoea, acute amoebic dysentery (proctocolitis with blood and mucus in the stool), chronic nondysenteric amoebiasis (diarrhoea, mucus, weight loss, and colonic ulceration), amoeboma (localized mass of granulation tissue), toxic megacolon, colonic stricture, and amoebic peritonitis. Extraintestinal manifestations include liver abscess (10%), and cutaneous or venereal amoebiasis. Hepatic abscesses may rupture into contiguous organs, such as the lung, pericardium, and inferior vena cava.

Physical examination

Patients may exhibit weight loss, fever, and dehydration. There may be tender hepatomegaly, upper abdominal distension, haematochezia, and leukocytes in the stool. Jaundice and peritonitis are uncommon.

Laboratory and special examinations

Typically, leukocytosis, anaemia, hypoalbuminaemia, elevated serum alkaline phosphatase, and elevated prothrombin time are present. Wet stool preparations (x3) (**291**) or endoscopic stool smears for trophozoites should be examined. Colonoscopy (without enemas or laxatives for preparation) shows haemorrhagic mucosa and discrete ulcers, typically with a shallow base and raised undermined edges. The disease may be limited to the rectum, caecum, or ascending colon. Biopsies from the edge of the ulcers may demonstrate *E. histolytica* (PAS stain). The antiamoebic antibody is of diagnostic value in amoebic liver abscess (sensitivity, **99%**) or amoebic dysentery (sensitivity, **88%**), but does not distinguish between previous or active infection. Imaging modalities (ultrasound, CT, MRI) are helpful in identifying liver abscess.

Differential diagnosis

Differentiate from inflammatory bowel disease, irritable colon syndrome, colitis due to other causes, and pyogenic liver abscess.

Prognosis

Fulminant colitis or liver abscess may prove fatal (**292**). Amoebiasis is most severe in the malnourished, young, elderly, pregnant, or immunosuppressed (20–30% case fatality rates).

Management

Invasive colonic disease and liver abscess are treated by metronidazole for 10 days. Liver abscess may also be treated by a combination of metronidazole and chloroquine. More toxic drugs include emetine and dihydroemetine. Percutaneous aspiration is necessary only for liver abscesses with impending rupture. Surgery is rarely indicated. Asymptomatic cyst passers may be treated by diloxanide furoate, iodoquinol, or paromomycin, although reinfection is frequent in endemic areas.

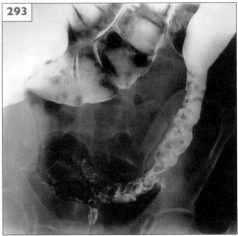

292 Postmortem liver showing amoebic abscess.

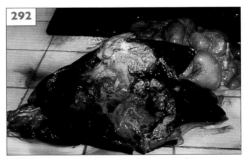

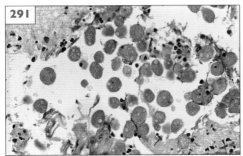

291 Stool examination shows the presence of round amoebae, which have ingested red cells, showing that they are pathogenic.

293 Narrowed irregular colonic appearances in a patient with schistosomiasis on barium enema.

SCHISTOSOMIASIS
Epidemiology and aetiology
Schistosomiasis (*Schistosoma mansoni*) is widespread in Africa, Latin America and the Middle East. *S. japonicum* is prevalent in the Far East, including China, Japan, the Philippines and Indochina. Humans serve as the definitive host. The ova are excreted in the stools, and hatch into miracidia upon reaching fresh water. Further development into cercariae occurs in freshwater snails. Through human water-related activities, cercariae gain access to the skin, enter the body, and mature into adult worms in the superior mesenteric vein (*S. mansoni*) or inferior mesenteric vein (*S. japonicum*). *S. haematobium* live in the vesical plexus and only rarely cause gastrointestinal complications. The worms live their life as pairs, with the female living inside the male within venules, and release 301–3,500 eggs daily. Lytic enzymes produced by the ova facilitate penetration by the worm of the venule wall and entry into the intestinal lumen.

Pathophysiology
The cutaneous migration of larvae excites local inflammation (cutaneous larva migrans). Deposition of ova into the portal vein or the intestinal wall leads to chronic inflammation and fibrosis. The eventual consequences depend upon the worm burden, as well as the host immune response.

Clinical history
Cutaneous larva migrans may be asymptomatic or excite mild pruritic dermatitis. Visceral larva migrans may be associated with fever, urticaria, serum sickness-like illness, cough, weight loss, and eosinophilia. Colonic schistosomiasis may cause abdominal pain, diarrhoea, and blood in the stool. Strictures (**293**) or polyps may occur. Periportal liver fibrosis causes portal hypertension, hepatosplenomegaly, variceal bleeding, and ascites with a relatively preserved hepatic parenchymal function. Portasystemic shunting of eggs to the lungs may cause chronic pulmonary hypertension and cor pulmonale.

Physical examination
Typical findings in advanced cases are hepatosplenomegaly, ascites, or prominent abdominal collateral veins. Early cases may show no abnormal signs.

Laboratory and special examinations
Investigations are for ova in the stool (**294**), and rectal or liver biopsy (**295**). Direct smears have a low sensitivity. Colonoscopy may demonstrate diffuse or patchy erythema, friability, and 'schistosomal polyps' containing eggs and granulation tissue. Serologic tests may be suggestive, but are not diagnostic.

Differential diagnosis
Differentiate from other causes of portal hypertension, diarrhoea, abdominal pain, and rectal bleeding.

Prognosis
The course is indolent, and eradication of the worms has generally been difficult. Coinfection with either hepatitis B or C markedly accelerates liver disease. If fatal, patients usually die of liver disease.

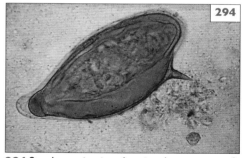

294 Stool examination showing the presence of a schistosome; the laterally placed spike shows that it is *S. mansoni.*

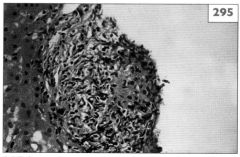

295 A granuloma in the liver of a patient with schistosomiasis.

Management

Praziquantel kills the worms and is indicated for all patients. Oxamniquine is an alternative for *S. mansoni*. However, eradication of the worms may not reverse the disease. Symptomatic treatments are necessary for gastrointestinal bleeding, ascites, and heart failure. The development of a vaccine is being actively pursued.

CHAGAS' DISEASE

Epidemiology and aetiology

Chagas' disease (caused by *Trypanosoma cruzi*) afflicts millions in Latin America, with thousands of deaths annually. The parasite is transmitted from infected humans or animals by the reduvid bug, with circulating trypomastigotes. Metacyclic trypomastigotes develop in the insect intestines, and enter humans through contamination of insect bites with infected insect faeces.

Pathophysiology

The host genetics, parasite factors, and autoimmune responses involved in disease pathogenesis are incompletely defined. Myocardial destruction and fibrosis is characteristic, and the myenteric plexus in the gastrointestinal tract is destroyed with abnormal gut hormone responses.

Clinical history

Acute infections are usually asymptomatic, although periorbital oedema at the site of the reduvid bug bite, fever, adenopathy, hepatosplenomegaly, or myocarditis may be noted. Chronic infection manifests years later with cardiac or gastrointestinal disease. Cardiac arrhythmias, cardiomyopathy, dysphagia, regurgitation, and constipation are typical.

Physical examination

Patients should be examined for cardiomegaly, megaoesophagus, and megacolon.

Laboratory and special examinations

This includes taking Giemsa-stained smears from tissues, cultivating the organisms in special media, PCR, and serological tests. Analysis of reduvid bugs may help. Chest radiograph, plain radiograph of the abdomen, and barium studies of the oesophagus and colon are helpful.

Differential diagnosis

Differentiate from a variety of gastrointestinal disorders causing neuromuscular disease, including myopathies, autonomic neuropathy, progressive systemic sclerosis, Hirschsprung's disease, and drug-induced pseudo-obstruction (narcotics, laxative abuse, antidepressants, etc.).

Prognosis

The natural history is of progressive deterioration and death due to cardiac complications.

Management

Only symptomatic treatments are available. Specific antiprotozoal therapies are available for acute infection.

ENTEROBIUS VERMICULARIS (PINWORM)

Epidemiology and aetiology

This is a parasitic worm endemic in temperate and tropical climates. Schoolchildren are most frequently affected. Poor personal hygiene is usually incriminated. The transmission is by ingestion of ova, which hatch in the upper small bowel and mature during transit through the ileum. The adult worms live in the distal colon.

Pathophysiology

The female migrates through the anus to lay eggs in perianal or perineal skin, which leads to local symptoms.

Clinical history

If symptomatic, there is perianal skin irritation, pruritus ani, vulvovaginitis, and occasionally granulomatous peritonitis (migration of worms through the colonic wall or female genital tract).

Physical examination

Patients should be examined for perianal erythema or secondary infection.

Laboratory and special examinations

This is by microscopic examination of worms picked up on adhesive cellophane tape applied to the anal region (sensitivity of three smears, 90%). Identification of stool ova and parasites is less sensitive (10–15%).

Differential diagnosis
Differentiate from other worm infections.

Prognosis
Worm eradication requires improved personal hygiene, treatment of other family members, and thorough decontamination of bedlinen and personal clothing.

Management
Mebendazole, albendazole, and pyrantel pamoate are effective wormicidal agents.

TRICHURIS TRICHURIA (WHIPWORM)
Epidemiology and aetiology
This parasite is prevalent in the tropics. Infection occurs by contact with contaminated stools. After ingestion of embryonated eggs, the larvae excyst and penetrate the intestinal mucosa with their thread-like anterior ends, moult, mature, and reattach as adults to the caecal or colonic mucosa. The mature females release 2,000–6,000 eggs daily. The maturation of eggs requires 10–14 days in the soil.

Pathophysiology
Symptoms depend upon the worm burden, and are due to mechanical or parasitic phenomena. Children are most commonly affected.

Clinical history
Presentation ranges from asymptomatic states to anaemia, growth retardation, and bloody or mucoid stools. Rectal prolapse, and colonic obstruction or perforation, are rare.

Physical examination
Physical examination is not helpful.

Laboratory and special examinations
This involves monitoring eosinophilia, ova in the stools, and worms in the colonic mucosa (**296**).

Differential diagnosis
Differentiate from other parasitic infestations.

Prognosis
Prognosis is usually excellent.

Management
Worms are eradicated by mebendazole or albendazole. In addition, public health measures should be taken (sanitary stool disposal, hand washing, and thorough cleaning and cooking of food).

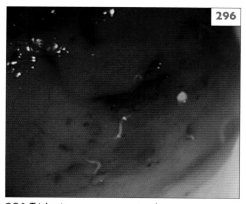

296 *Trichuria* worms seen at colonoscopy.

Diverticular disease of the colon

Definition
Colonic diverticula represent bowel wall projections, which create extraluminal pouches. Diverticulitis results from inflammatory exacerbations, due to impacted materials in the diverticula.

Epidemiology and aetiology
The prevalence is far greater in industrialized societies, particularly in the West, ranging from 5 to 45% of the population. There is an age-dependent increase in the prevalence of colonic diverticula, which may exceed 50% in people aged over 80 years. They are rarely found before age 40. In Western societies, changes in dietary fibre intake and switching to low-residue diets are believed to account for increased prevalence. Diverticular disease is rare in agrarian societies with high dietary fibre intake, such as in Africa and India. Whether additional host-specific factors contribute is unclear.

Pathophysiology
The diverticula arise in the colon, where colonic arteries penetrate the muscularis to reach the mucosa (**297**). The diverticula lack muscularis mucosa and are of pulsion type, probably related to prolonged straining at stool and excessively increased intracolonic pressures. Diverticula are mostly in the sigmoid and the left-sided colon (95%), less frequently in the ascending, transverse, and descending colon (35%), and least often throughout the colon (7%).

Complications
Diverticulitis develops when the mouth of a diverticulum becomes impacted by faecal material, followed by infection and erosion through the serosa, leakage or perforation, and development of a localized inflammatory mass. Erosion into a blood vessel may produce profuse haemorrhage, although this is uncommon.

Clinical history
Most cases of diverticulosis are asymptomatic (70%). Clinical manifestations are of the complications:
- Diverticulitis (10–25%) presents with subacute left lower quadrant pain, fever, and constipation or loose stools.
- Rectal haemorrhage (5%) is infrequent.

Physical examination
In the absence of complications, there are no abnormal signs. In the presence of diverticulitis, typical findings are tachycardia, fever, and tenderness, distension, or a mass in the left lower quadrant.

Laboratory and special examinations
Laboratory findings include leukocytosis and mild anaemia with diverticulitis. A plain radiograph of the abdomen may demonstrate air beneath the diaphragm, or extraluminal gas if bowel perforation has occurred. A colonoscopy may be helpful in distinguishing from colitis or cancer, but is relatively contraindicated in acute diverticulitis (**298**). CT is useful for assessing bowel thickening, local inflammatory collection, or liver abscess formation (**299**). A barium enema may demonstrate mucosal irregularities and bowel spasm, perforation, abscess, or fistula formation (**300**).

Differential diagnosis
Differentiate from inflammatory bowel disease, bacterial colitis, ischaemic bowel disease, irritable colon syndrome, colon cancer, and gynaecological disorders, e.g. salpingo-oophoritis. Remember that diverticulosis is common and may coexist with these conditions.

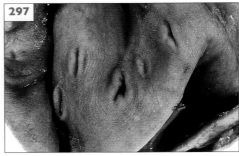

297 A resection specimen showing colonic diverticula from the luminal side.

Prognosis

Patients may remain asymptomatic throughout life, or have only minimal symptoms. Severe diverticulitis may require surgical intervention. Bleeding may be paroxysmal and life-threatening. Complications include colonic stricture, perforation, abscess, fistulous communications with adjacent organs (including bladder and small intestine), and septicaemia.

Management

Diverticulitis is treated with antibiotics (third-generation cephalosporin plus metronidazole), intravenous fluids, and bowel rest for several days. Abscesses may be drained percutaneously. Unremitting disease may require surgical intervention and hemicolectomy, debridement, or additional measures. Increased dietary fibre intake, stool softeners, and avoidance of constipation help in decreasing symptoms of diverticular disease.

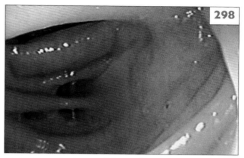

298 Diverticulosis of the colon at endoscopy.

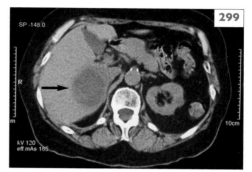

299 Complicated diverticular disease. CT showing liver abscess, secondary to infection through portal circulation.

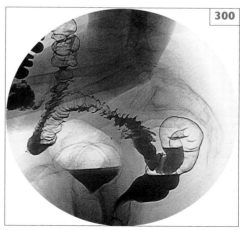

300 Complicated diverticular disease, with a fistula well demonstrated between the sigmoid colon and the bladder.

Hirschsprung's disease and congenital megacolon

Definition
This is a developmental disorder characterized by defective neural crest cell migration during colonic development, leading to an 'aganglionic' segment.

Epidemiology and aetiology
Genetic mutations have been identified with autosomal recessive (chromosome 13) and autosomal dominant (chromosome 10) transmission. The disorder is relatively uncommon and may come to diagnosis in neonates, early childhood, or adult life.

Pathophysiology
The aganglionic segment of the colon causes a functional obstruction due to a failure to relax. The proximal bowel is hypertrophied and dilated. The rectosigmoid region is most frequently affected (75–80%), although the entire colon and variable lengths of the small bowel may be affected (5–10%). The affected segment is usually very short in adults.

Clinical history
- In the newborn: there is delayed passage of meconium and abdominal distension.
- In children: there is chronic constipation, abdominal distension, volvulus, or perforation.
- In adults: there is chronic constipation from childhood, or dramatic intermittent constipation.

Physical examination
A rectal examination shows an empty rectal vault in Hirschsprung's disease. By contrast, stool is present in idiopathic megacolon.

Laboratory and special examinations
Plain radiograph of the abdomen shows colonic dilatation and a paucity of gas in the rectum. A barium enema shows a short, narrow segment or transition zone (**301**) and may be normal. Anal manometry demonstrates failure of the internal sphincter to relax in response to rectal distension. Histology using a full-thickness biopsy is usually necessary for diagnosis. The most typical feature is absence of ganglion cells in the submucosa and myenteric plexus, identification of which is facilitated by acetylcholinesterase staining.

Differential diagnosis
Differentiate from other structural and congenital abnormalities (intestinal duplications, malrotation, imperforate anus, volvulus), Chagas' disease, and other causes of colonic dilatation.

Prognosis
Prognosis is usually good.

Management
Treatment is surgical. Neonates may require a colostomy or pull-through of the bowel to the anus. In short-segment aganglionosis, rectal myectomy alone may be adequate.

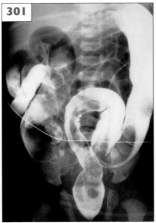

301 Barium enema in Hirschsprung's disease in a newborn, showing a short, narrow segment or transition zone and dilated colon above.

Solitary rectal ulcer

Definition
This is nonspecific ulceration of the rectum, with characteristic disorganization of the muscularis mucosa.

Epidemiology and aetiology
The disorder is infrequent and tends to affect young adults – females more than males. It usually appears in the third or the fourth decade of life, although the age range is wider (10–80 years). Chronic constipation and straining at stool, as well as rectal injury during manual stool evacuation, may be involved.

Pathophysiology
The precise chain of events has not been reproduced. It is thought that straining and excessive voiding pressure during stool evacuation may produce rectal prolapse, functional ischaemia, and ulceration. Local trauma may play a role.

Clinical history
Constipation, tenesmus, straining at stool, and lower abdominal pain are frequent (70–90%). Mild rectal bleeding may occur (50–90% of cases) but profuse rectal bleeding is highly unusual. One-quarter of the patients are asymptomatic.

Physical examination
Rectal induration or bleeding may be apparent on digital examination. The ulcers are usually within a few centimetres of the anal verge, and may affect the anterior or posterior rectal wall.

Laboratory and special examinations
Iron-deficiency anaemia may be found. Unless carefully sought, the ulcers may be missed on flexible sigmoidoscopy (**302**). In view of the distal location, proctoscopy may be superior in visualization of a solitary rectal ulcer. Ulcers are shallow, but with an indurated edge. Usually, they occur close to the anus, and polypoid or mass lesions are sometimes seen. Biopsies from the edge of the ulcer demonstrate replacement of the lamina propria by fibroblasts, smooth muscle, and collagen. There is associated hypertrophy and disorganization of the muscularis mucosa, displacement of mucosal glands into the submucosa, and mucosal ulceration. The diffuse infiltration with collagen fibres is characteristic.

Differential diagnosis
Differentiate from Crohn's disease, ulcerative colitis, chronic ischaemic colitis, malignancy, venereal disease, and amoebiasis.

Prognosis
Prognosis is usually good.

Management
The mainstays are bulk laxatives, bowel retraining, and patient education. Surgery is reserved for refractory cases, excessive bleeding, or prolapse. Local excision, rectopexy, or (rarely) diverting colostomy may be performed.

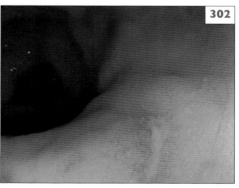

302 Solitary rectal ulcer syndrome, here seen as an ulcer. It can present a more polypoid form.

Vascular disorders of the bowel

Disruption to the vascular supply to the bowel leads to ischaemia (disease of the small bowel is considered in Chapter 5). The vascular process affecting the coeliac axis, superior mesenteric, or inferior mesenteric circulation may be occlusive, nonocclusive, or a combination of these. Whether the colon suffers ischaemic damage depends upon the state of the general circulation, collateral blood flow, response to autonomic stimuli, release of circulating vasoactive substances, and local modulation of blood flow. Different clinical scenarios are colonic ischaemia (60%) or acute mesenteric ischaemia affecting the small intestine (30%) and, less often, chronic mesenteric ischaemia (5%) or focal segmental ischaemia (5%). Colonic angiodysplasia, telangiectasia, or portasystemic varices constitute additional vascular disorders.

ISCHAEMIC COLITIS
Definition
Ischaemic colitis is defined as colonic injury due to interrupted blood supply.

Epidemiology and aetiology
The colon may be affected by superior mesenteric artery disease (50% occlusion, 25% ischaemia, 10% thrombosis) in the setting of left atrial or ventricular thrombosis, acute myocardial infarction, congestive heart failure, arrhythmias and shock; thrombosis of the superior mesenteric vein due to hypercoagulative states, coagulation disorders, polycythaemia vera or oestrogen excess; and by focal segmental ischaemia (10%) from emboli, vasculitis, radiation, trauma, intestinal obstruction, enteritis, hernia, etc. Isolated colonic ischaemia mostly affects patients aged over 60 years (90%) – in this setting, no apparent cause may be found at presentation. Younger individuals may present with colonic injury due to vasculitis, sickle cell disease, coagulopathies, drugs (such as cocaine), and occasionally long-distance running.

Pathophysiology
Simultaneous involvement of the small and large gut in ischaemic injury (coeliac or superior mesenteric artery occlusion) is devastating, with mortality rates approaching 90% in the presence of peritonitis. Involvement of the colon alone most frequently causes reversible submucosal or intramural haemorrhage (30–40%), transient necrosis (15–20%), gangrene (15–20%), chronic ulceration (20–25%), or stricture (10–15%), and less often fulminant necrosis (approximately 5%). The systemic manifestations are related to perfusion-reperfusion injury, and release of vasoactive substances or inflammatory mediators. The histological correlates of acute ischaemic colitis are extensive haemorrhage, congestion, oedema (**303**), and necrosis with or without perforation, gangrene, and stricture. Although any part of the colon may be affected, the splenic flexure, descending colon, and sigmoid colon are most often involved in acute ischaemic colitis.

Clinical history
There is sudden cramping left lower abdominal pain, tenesmus, and bright red or maroon blood per rectum. Acute mesenteric ischaemia may be 'silent', and patients can present with shock, confusion, or metabolic acidosis.

Physical examination
Typically, there are diminished or absent bowel sounds, lower abdominal tenderness, and signs of peritonitis or bowel perforation.

Laboratory and special examinations
Anticipated finding include leukocytosis, anaemia, metabolic acidosis, and elevated serum amylase, lactate dehydrogenase, and creatine phosphokinase. A plain radiograph of the abdomen may show colonic intramural oedema or haemorrhage producing 'thumb-printing', as well as free air in the peritoneal cavity. Colonoscopy or flexible sigmoidoscopy may show extensive mucosal haemorrhage, and congestion or ulceration (**304**). A barium enema may interfere with subsequent angiography. Visceral angiography can demonstrate site of occlusion. Investigate also for occult pro-coagulant disorders (eg anti-cardiolipin antibodies, JAK-2 mutations, pro-coagulant screens).

Differential diagnosis
Differentiate from inflammatory bowel disease, infectious colitis, radiation colitis, and the various causes of acute abdomen.

Prognosis
Acute mesenteric ischaemia is fatal in 40–50% of cases, with mortality rates approaching 90% in the presence of generalized peritonitis –

indicating bowel perforation (**305–307**). In isolated colonic involvement, the prognosis is better with only submucosal or intramural haemorrhage in two-thirds, and transient colitis in one-third. Irreversible colonic injury occurs in 50% of cases, however. Patients may re-present with a delayed stricture 4–6 weeks after an initial acute presentation with diarrhoea and bleeding.

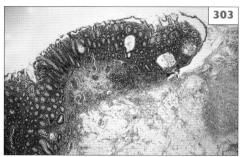

303 Histopathological section showing swollen congested mucosa with loss of epithelial cells in ischaemic colitis.

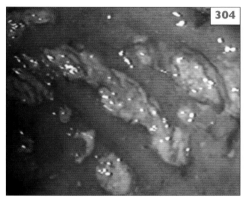

304 'Punched-out' ulcers seen at colonoscopy in a patient with ischaemic colitis.

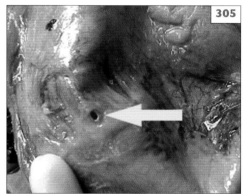

305 Caecal perforation in a patient with ischaemic colitis.

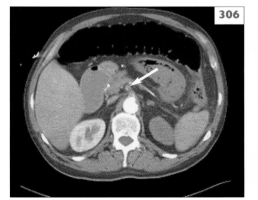

306 CT scan showing thrombosis of the superior mesenteric artery in a patient with aortic dissection (left kidney also not perfused)

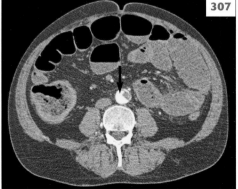

307 Thrombosis of the superior mesenteric artery showing dilated and secondary ischaemic bowel.

Management

Patients with severe disease require aggressive resuscitation and intensive care, broad-spectrum antibiotics, and surgery. An underlying cause should be sought. In the absence of perforation or gangrene, patients may be managed by bowel rest, antibiotics, and sometimes short-term anticoagulation.

COLONIC ANGIODYSPLASIA

Definition

Vascular ectasias affect the colonic mucosa in the absence of cutaneous lesions, systemic disease, or a familial syndrome.

Epidemiology and aetiology

Prospective studies are necessary to determine the true prevalence. Asymptomatic angiodysplasia is frequent and may be found in 3–6% of cases at colonoscopy. Angiodysplasia can occur in various sites throughout the gastrointestinal tract, in addition to the colon, and can be the source of occult gastrointestinal bleeding and iron-deficiency anaemia. Colonic angiodysplasia is one of the most common causes of recurrent gastrointestinal bleeding in the elderly. Most patients with symptoms are aged over 70 years, although some patients may present earlier. There is a loosely defined association of uncertain significance between colonic angiodysplasia and valvular aortic stenosis. Bleeding from angiodysplasia is also more common in patients with end-stage renal failure.

Pathophysiology

Angiodysplasia is most common in the caecum and ascending colon (**308**). Prominent dilated and tortuous submucosal veins are the earliest and most constant feature (**309**). The ectasias consist of dilated, thin-walled, distorted veins, venules, or capillaries lined by epithelium alone, or by variable amounts of smooth muscle. Most ectasias are <1 cm in diameter. More than one ectatic lesion is generally found.

Clinical history

There may be recurrent colonic blood loss in the elderly, with bright red or maroon-coloured blood. Massive bleeding is uncommon (<15% of cases). Bleeding tends to stop by itself (90%). However, anaemia due to chronic occult bleeding may be the presenting manifestation.

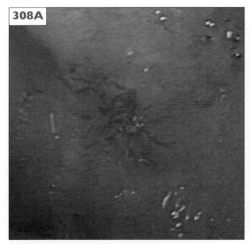 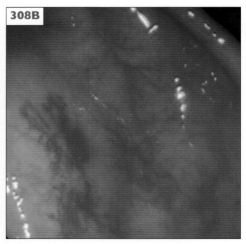

308 Two pictures of angioectasia as seen at colonoscopy.

Other, more florid, angiomatous malformations may give a similar clinical picture.

Physical examination
Typical findings are anaemia and cardiac lesions, and atherosclerotic peripheral vascular disease in some cases.

Laboratory and special examinations
Iron-deficiency anaemia should be looked for. Colonoscopy by the inexperienced may lead to overdiagnosis of angiodysplasia (sensitivity >80%). Total colonoscopy with good visualization of the caecum is necessary to exclude angiodysplasia. Angiography is diagnostic when one of the following is seen: dilated and slowly emptying vein within the bowel wall, arterial 'tufting' pattern, or an early filling vein during the arterial phase. Identification of the lesions in pathology specimens requires special techniques, such as instillation of barium or polymers in the vessels.

Differential diagnosis
Differentiate from malignancy, diverticular disease, and ischaemic colitis.

Prognosis
The course is usually indolent. Many patients remain asymptomatic throughout life. In 50% of patients, bleeding may be intermittent over 1–2 years.

Management
Treatment of bleeding angioectasia is usually conservative in view of advanced age, associated disorders, and rebleeding in only some patients. Endoscopic ablation of lesions by cautery, heat argon-plasma coagulation, or laser is often successful. The lesions can also be controlled by angiographic embolization, but there is a risk of inducing colonic ischaemia. Surgical resection may be necessary. Oestrogen-progesterone combinations have occasionally been beneficial. Asymptomatic and nonbleeding lesions found incidentally during investigation for other symptoms need not be treated.

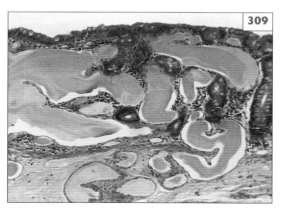

309 Injected histopathological specimen (light-pink injectate) showing dilated vascular spaces in the submucosa in caecal angiodysplasia.

Haemorrhoids, anal fissures, and fistulae

The venous plexus of vessels around the anorectal junction helps form a mucosal-covered cushion that aids continence. Haemorrhoids ('piles' in the vernacular) develop from congestion of venous plexuses, with associated mucosal hypertrophy and development of adjacent perirectal skin tags (**310**). In the more severe cases, parts of the venous plexus with the overlying mucosa prolapse from the rectum either intermittently or permanently.

Symptoms
Various symptoms are identified. Perianal itching may be associated with haemorrhoids; bleeding is the most common symptom leading patients to seek medical attention. Characteristically, there is bright red on the surface of the stool and on the lavatory paper, but not mixed with the stools. Thrombosis of external piles leads to a painful, hard, round lesion.

Management
Avoidance measures
- Prevention of straining at stool, passage of soft stool.

Treatment
- Maintenance of bowel habit as above.
- Bleeding may be treated by local sclerosis, or larger piles by ligation and banding surgically.
- Anal dilatation (under anaesthesia) may be used.

ACUTE ANAL FISSURES
This appears as a split in the surface epithelium of the anorectal junction, and causes substantial pain, particularly during defaecation. It is particularly likely to occur with severe constipation.

Management
Two approaches are possible:
- In the short term, dilatation of the rectum to allow stretching of the anal rectal sphincter, and to help initiate healing of the mucosa.
- In the long term, treatment of the constipation to allow regular passage of soft stool (as internal dilator); a high fibre intake helps.

ANAL FISTULA
Perianal fistula
Fistulous tracks may develop from the anal canal or the rectum, commencing as sinuses and tracking into the perianal tissue; in some instances, the tracks open out on to the perianal skin. Infection within these fistulous tracks causes both abscesses and persistent discharge from fistulous openings. Low fistulae open below the internal anal sphincter, and high fistulae open above. Complex fistulae are often associated with Crohn's disease (**311**). MRI can allow fistulous tracts to be imaged in great detail (**312**). The symptoms are those of pain and discharge. Treatment varies from antibiotics alone, release of pus under pressure, and, in persistent cases, local surgical treatment to lay fistulae open and allow healing with obliteration of the tract.

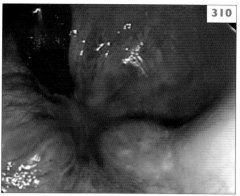

310 Retroflexed view in the rectum showing normal rectal mucosa, but haemorrhoids around the anal margin.

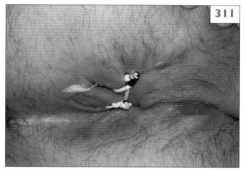

311 Extensive perianal involvement (abscesses and fistulae) in Crohn's disease. Setons are *in situ*.

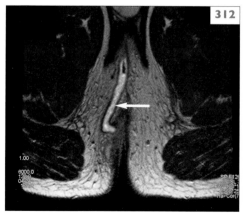

312 MRI demonstrating (arrowed) a perianal fistula and perianal abscess formation.

CHAPTER 9

Gastrointestinal bleeding

Acute gastrointestinal bleeding is a medical emergency. Endoscopy provides therapeutic as well as diagnostic opportunity

The source of obscure gastrointestinal bleeding may be elucidated by angiography, by capsule endoscopy, or by isotope scanning techniques

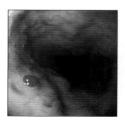 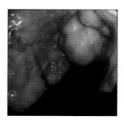 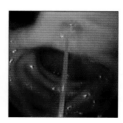 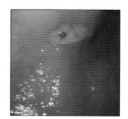

Introduction

Loss of blood from the gastrointestinal tract can be classified according to the site and type of haemorrhage, and the rate of bleeding. Gastrointestinal bleeding occurs predominantly from the upper tract (oesophagus, stomach, or duodenum), but also the lower tract (small intestine or colon). Bleeding can be acute or chronic. Chronic bleeding can be apparent or inapparent; in the latter case, presentation is with anaemia of the iron-deficiency type.

Symptoms
Acute upper gastrointestinal bleeding
This is characterized by haematemesis (vomiting of bright red blood) or 'coffee grounds' (blood denatured by gastric acid), melaena (dark tarry stools), or a combination. Oesophageal bleeding may be frank red, while gastric and duodenal bleeding tend to present with coffee grounds. Gastric and, in particular duodenal, bleeding may present with melaena only.

Acute lower gastrointestinal bleeding
Bleeding from haemorrhoids and the left side of the colon may be bright red and/or only slightly dark. Bleeding from the right side of the colon or distal terminal ileum tends to be maroon in colour. Bleeding from colitis is mixed with stool, but blood from vascular anomalies, Meckel's diverticulum, or diverticulae is often separate.

It is sometimes unclear on clinical grounds whether the bleeding is from the upper or lower gastrointestinal tract.

General management and diagnosis
Management and diagnosis of acute bleeding are interrelated.
- Assess severity of blood loss. Close monitoring of haemodynamic parameters (pulse, jugular venous pressure, central venous pressure, and urine output).
- Resuscitate with colloid, and transfuse blood as appropriate. Always arrange crossmatch.
- Endoscopy (emergency if bleeding severe, or on next available list if less severe). Early endoscopy identifies low-risk patients who can be discharged promptly, detects patients with a high risk of rebleeding who require continued close observation, and allows therapeutic intervention.

- Consider the range of therapeutic options (conservative/transfuse, interventional endoscopy, e.g. sclerotherapy, use of drugs, surgery).
- If emergency endoscopy does not diagnose source/cause of bleeding, and bleeding persists, consider alternative diagnostic techniques – red cell scanning, angiography, laparotomy.

Acute upper gastrointestinal bleeding

Typical causes include:
- Oesophageal varices.
- Mallory–Weiss tear.
- Oesophagitis.
- Gastric erosions.
- Gastric ulcer.
- Gastric cancer.
- Duodenal ulcer.
- Duodenal erosions.
- Miscellaneous.

Treatment
Gastrointestinal bleeding may stop spontaneously, but if there is persistent or severe bleeding, active intervention is required, whether endoscopic, surgical, or pharmacological in nature. If urgent intervention is not used, later treatment is often necessary to treat the underlying disease (e.g. heal duodenal ulceration). If there is persistent acute blood loss (>4 units of blood), particularly in the elderly, the chances of surgery being needed increase greatly.

OESOPHAGEAL VARICES
These comprise veins carrying blood from the high-pressure portal system to the systemic circulation, via the lower oesophagus (see Chapter 3). They are almost always a manifestation of portal hypertension and associated with underlying liver cirrhosis. Bleeding oesophageal varices are the most dangerous form of upper gastrointestinal bleeding, as there is often associated liver failure, including coagulopathy.

The diagnosis is usually made at endoscopy, when varices are seen as dilated varicose vessels in the lower third of the oesophagus (**313**). Other endoscopic findings in portal hypertension are associated varices in the stomach (**314**) or a general congestion of the stomach (portal gastropathy) (**315**).

Treatment of bleeding oesophageal varices

Treating shock with transfusion of blood and/or colloid is the priority. Sepsis is frequently a precipitant of bleeding and should be sorted; blind antibiotic treatment is appropriate.

Endoscopic therapy

Active oesophageal bleeding can be arrested by various endoscopic therapies, including:
- Band ligation of the bleeding varices by placing rubber bands, via the endoscope, onto the surface of the varices to obliterate them (see Chapter 3).
- Endoscopic injecting of sclerosant fluid into, or adjacent to, varices. This is an older technique but is sometimes technically easier in the setting of acute variceal bleeding. More recently, direct injection of 'tissue glues' has established a role in difficult-to-control variceal bleeding, particularly gastric varices.

Balloon tamponade
- Passage of multibore tubes with two inflatable balloons (Sengstaken–Blakemore tubes), which, when inflated, press against bleeding varices to stop bleeding as a temporizing measure.

Pharmacological intervention
- Intravenous terlipressin (a vasopressin analogue) to reduce portal pressure and aid cessation of haemorrhage. If terlipressin is not available, high-dose somatostatin may be of benefit.

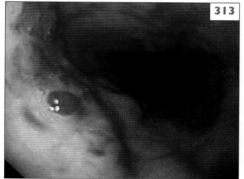

313 Oesophageal varices seen at endoscopy. A cherry red spot is seen — a feature associated with a high risk of bleeding.

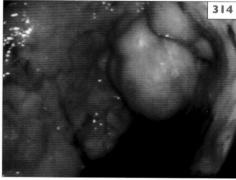

314 Gastric varices — these varices have recently bled, as there is altered blood in the stomach.

315 The 'snake skin' appearance of portal gastropathy.

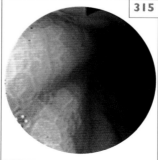

316 TIPSS — a tract between the hepatic and portal veins is established and then dilated (**A**) before a stent is placed (**B**).

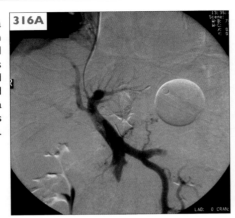
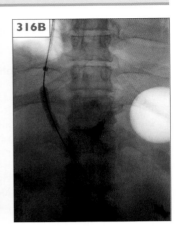

Radiological approaches

- Formation of a portal systemic shunt to decrease portal pressure by placing a stent from the hepatic vein through the substance of the liver to the portal vein (**316**). TIPSS reduces portal pressure and so controls bleeding but can cause deterioration in liver function and precipitate worsening encephalopathy.

Surgery

- A direct surgical approach to oversew the varices, or to disconnect bleeding varices from the portal circulation by oesophageal transection and reanastomosis. Surgical shunts are rarely required in the acute setting.

The treatment approach for each patient has to be individualized, as each technique has disadvantages. Sclerotherapy can induce ulceration in the distal oesophagus, and banding can be difficult during severe blood loss. Pharmacological treatment is often ineffective. Balloon tamponade may cause oesophageal trauma and aspiration pneumonia. The portal systemic shunt precipitates hepatic encephalopathy. Major surgery may be poorly tolerated.

MALLORY–WEISS TEAR

This is an acute tear at the oesophagogastric junction, which is initiated by retching/vomiting. There is a characteristic history of repeated vomiting – often after alcoholic binging – with vomiting of bright red blood after several episodes of vomiting without blood. Endoscopy shows gaping of mucosa, seen as a linear longitudinal tear at the oesophagogastric junction (**317**).

Treatment

The condition generally settles spontaneously, but endoscopic therapy is sometimes appropriate with localized endoscopic injection of sclerosants or dilute adrenaline (epinephrine).

Prognosis

Complete healing is anticipated.

ULCER BLEEDING

This occurs predominantly from duodenal or gastric ulcers. Both are diagnosed at endoscopy and treated if appropriate (**318-320**).

Management

Various clinical scoring systems have been developed to stratify risk. These are surrogate measures of blood loss and based on haemodynamic compensation, comorbidities, age, and endoscopic criteria. The prognosis of patients with upper gastrointestinal bleeding is poorer in the elderly, large volume bleeds, shock, hospital inpatients with bleeds, and patients with variceal bleeding.

Endoscopic criteria are the best predictor risk of recurrent bleeding. Rebleeding (and mortality) is highest in ulcers with spurting arterial vessels, followed by ulcers with nonbleeding visible vessels in the base, ulcers with adherent clots, pigmented flat lesions, and, finally, clean-based ulcers, which have a very low risk of rebleed.

317
Mallory–Weiss tear of the lower oesophagus: (**A**) from above; and (**B**) with the endoscope in the retroflexed 'J' position.

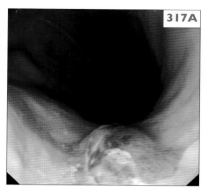

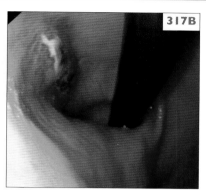

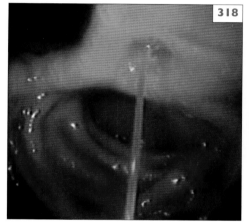

318 Peptic ulcer with arterial 'spurter'. This ulcer was successfully treated using the methods outlined in the text.

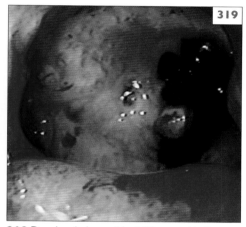

319 Duodenal ulcer with visible vessel in base.

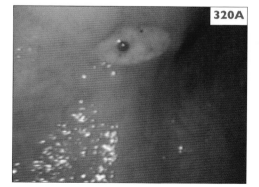

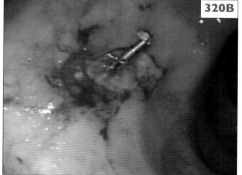

320 Endoscopic therapy to a gastric ulcer with visible vessel in the base (**A**). The ulcer area is injected in four quadrants and the base with dilute adrenaline (epinephrine), causing blanching of the mucosa. In (**B**), an endoclip is applied to the vessel.

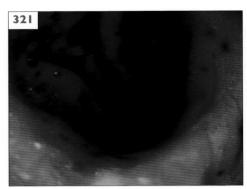

321 Haemorrhagic gastritis with multiple small areas of mucosal bleeding.

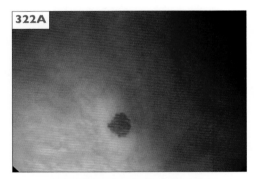

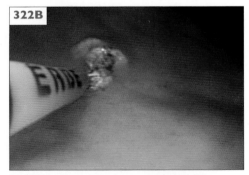

322 Telangiectasia in the stomach (**A**). These lesions are easily cauterized using argon-plasma coagulation – the probe is seen in (**B**).

Endotherapy of bleeding lesions

Endoscopic treatment of bleeding gastric and duodenal ulcer is evolving. The current best practice is to deliver therapy in two phases. Initially, the ulcer margin and base is injected with 10–20 ml of fluid, to promote tamponade of the bleeding vessel and local vasoconstriction. Usually, dilute adrenaline (epinephrine) is injected, but use of alcohol or other sclerosing fluids has been described. Secondly, the bleeding vessel should be physically coapted by a heater probe, diathermy, or endoscopic clipping device. Endotherapy is generally reserved for actively bleeding ulcers or those with high risk of recurrent bleeding (**319, 320**). With rebleeding, there should be a low threshold for surgery, particularly in the elderly.

Follow-up treatment

Treatment to heal ulcers should be started as soon as practicable, but does not alter the outcome of acute bleeding. Some studies show benefit from infusion of proton pump inhibitors for patients with bleeding peptic ulcers, following maximal endoscopic therapy.

GASTRIC EROSIONS

Diffuse loss of the mucosal epithelium and small ulcers can cause persistent haemorrhage (**321**). This condition is often associated with the use of NSAIDs and intake of alcohol. The condition is diagnosed at endoscopy, but treatment may be difficult. Conservative treatment includes a pharmacological approach to reduce splanchnic blood flow (e.g. somatostatin), multiple heat probing, or surgery.

MISCELLANEOUS

A simple gastric endartery bleed may cause severe bleeding (Dieulafoy's lesion). Small telangiectasias in the stomach or small intestine may bleed (**322**). These may be part of the autosomal dominant familial condition of hereditary haemorrhagic telangiectasia, in which case there may be similar lesions on the face (**323**). Occasionally, large congenital vascular abnormalities involve the small intestine; wireless capsule endoscopy has made it much easier to identify small vascular lesions in the small bowel (**324**).

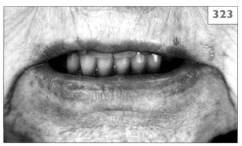

323 Small red telangiectasias seen around the lip (note upper lip), characteristic of Osler–Rendu–Weber hereditary haemorrhagic telangiectasia.

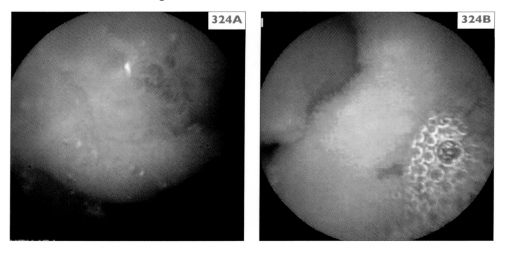

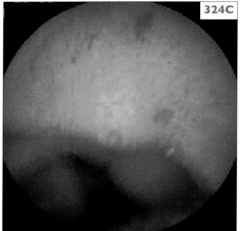

324 Three wireless capsule endoscopy images of small-bowel vascular lesions. Small lesions like this can be a cause of iron-deficiency anaemia.

Acute lower gastrointestinal bleeding

Lower gastrointestinal tract bleeding can present as an acute gastrointestinal bleed. Management is similar to an upper gastrointestinal bleed; the priority is restoration of haemodynamic stability with appropriate transfusion of blood and colloid. With upper gastrointestinal bleeding the ethos is early endoscopy to define the source and potentially treat the bleeding lesion. In the context of acute lower gastrointestinal bleeding, colonoscopy is frequently unrewarding, potentially hazardous, and so usually deferred until the bleeding has stopped.

DIVERTICULAR DISEASE

Bleeding from colonic diverticula can present with sudden painless and rapid loss of frank blood from dilated veins in sigmoid colonic diverticula – blood loss can exceed 500 ml or more (**325, 326**). Typically, the patient is elderly. Acute diagnosis is by urgent colonoscopy. However, this is often difficult in the unprepared colon, and so diagnosis may be presumptive when subsequent elective colonoscopy/barium enema shows diverticula. Surgery is rarely indicated. Usually, bleeding stops spontaneously but it can recur in up to one-third of patients. Follow-up treatment is generally conservative; a high-roughage diet may be indicated for diverticulosis.

RECTAL/COLONIC POLYPS

This is seen as intermediate loss of small volumes of blood – often occult – and frequently presents as iron-deficiency anaemia. Diagnosis is by colonoscopy/barium enema in a prepared colon. Colonoscopy offers the opportunity for polypectomy (and therefore also cancer prevention by removal of preneoplastic lesions).

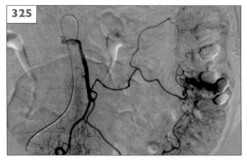

325 Inferior mesenteric arteriogram of a bleed in the descending colon. This was due to a bleeding diverticulum.

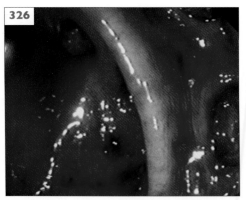

326 Diverticulosis, seen in the setting of a recent rectal bleed.

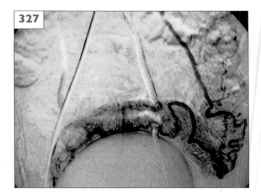

327 Inferior mesenteric angiogram showing gross arterial and venous abnormalities in the sigmoid colon (haemangioma).

ANGIODYSPLASIA

This is an abnormal vasculature developing in the colon; it is predominantly caecal and more common with advancing age. There are dilated ectatic submucosal blood vessels, with both arterial and venous ectasia. The condition presents with intermittent blood loss – either visible (often dark red) – or with iron-deficiency anaemia. For acute diagnosis, the condition is usually invisible on barium enema, but may be diagnosed by colonoscopy (with difficulty in an unprepared colon) or by angiography (see below).

For treatment, use colonoscopic diathermy for electrocoagulation of lesions, argon-plasma coagulation, or resection of the affected area.

Haemangiomas are more extensive abnormalities, which can present in a similar way (**327**).

COLONIC CANCER

If bleeding, this condition presents with symptoms similar to those of a rectal polyp. Severe bleeding occurs only rarely. Right-sided lesions classically present with iron-deficiency anaemia. Diagnosis is by colonoscopy or barium enema. Treatment is with surgical resection.

ISCHAEMIC COLITIS

The ischaemic colitides are considered in Chapter 8. The diagnosis should be considered in elderly patients presenting with dark red bleeding, mixed with the stools, and is often associated with pain. Diagnosis is sometimes suggested by plain abdominal radiograph or CT scan, which may show oedema or 'thumb-printing' of ischaemic colon. Treatment is generally conservative, as the colitis generally resolves. However, an underlying cause should be sought. Some patients are offered short-term anticoagulation. Later consequences may include stricture, which occasionally requires resection.

OTHER CAUSES

Ulcerative colitis and bacillary dysentery both cause rectal bleeding, but this is part of an exudative diarrhoea, with pus, mucus, and tenesmus. Colonic Crohn's disease can rarely present with a gastrointestinal bleed.

Haemorrhoidal bleeding has the characteristics of oozing postdefaecation (bright red blood), often after passage of hard stools. Blood is only often noticed on the toilet paper or in the lavatory pan. Such blood loss is only very rarely sufficient to cause anaemia.

Gastrointestinal bleeding: some general points

In obscure/recurrent gastrointestinal bleeding – which remains undiagnosed after routine endoscopy and radiograph of the upper and lower gastrointestinal tract – the following should be considered:

- Wireless capsule endoscopy.
- Visceral angiography.
- Red cell scanning.
- Exploratory laparotomy.

Angiography may show an abnormality, which can potentially bleed (e.g. angiodysplasia of the caecum). In acute bleeding, blood loss can be demonstrated actively by leakages of contrast medium into the bowel lumen if the blood loss is more than 0.5–1 ml/min.

Super-selective angiography can sometimes identify specific bleeding vessels, with the opportunity to embolize these vessels with coils, etc. The procedure can be used in both acute and chronic bleeding (**328, 329**).

Red cell scanning using tagged red cells can indicate bleeding at rates of less than 0.5 ml/min. It lacks the diagnostic accuracy of angiography and has no therapeutic capability. However, it can occasionally be helpful in directing surgeons to the appropriate bowel region.

In young patients, most causes of obscure gastrointestinal bleeding would be readily found by the surgeon at laparotomy (e.g. Meckel's diverticulum or tumours). In elderly patients, vascular anomalies are the dominant cause of bleeding, and routine laparotomy does not demonstrate this. Specialized techniques, such as on-table total endoscopy with transillumination of the bowel, may help to show vascular anomalies at surgery.

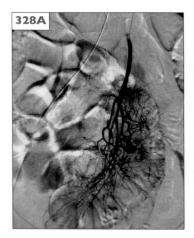
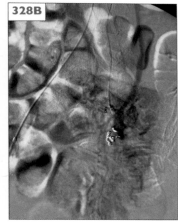

328 Two views of a selective visceral angiogram in a patient with recurrent acute gastrointestinal bleeds. The bleeding is from an abnormal leash of vessels (**A**), which were successfully embolized (**B**).

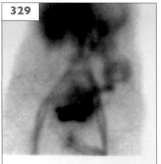

329 Red cell scan from a patient with obscure gastrointestinal bleeding: Tracer is seen in the left upper quadrant, indicating bleeding in the upper part of the small intestine.

Small-intestinal bleeding

MECKEL'S DIVERTICULUM

This is a remnant of the embryonic vitellointestinal duct, situated 60 cm from the ileocaecal valve (**330–332**). It is the cause of intermittent blood loss, which is seen as a deep maroon-coloured stool, and may be associated with a history of postprandial pain. The condition is caused by ulceration of the ectopic gastric mucosa in the diverticulum. Meckel's scan (^{99m}Tc scanning) may show excretion of the isotope by the ectopic gastric mucosa, but is not reliable.

Other causes

Other causes of small-intestinal bleeding have been identified. Although rare, these include:
- Ulcers induced by NSAIDs.
- Tumours – carcinoma, lymphoma, leiomyoma (tumour of smooth muscle).
- Vascular anomalies (haemangioma, angiodysplasia). Blood loss may be obvious (generally melaena-like) or inapparent (in which case presentation is with iron-deficiency anaemia).

Diagnosis

This is often difficult because:
- Small-intestinal causes of blood loss are often not considered.
- Such problems are generally beyond the reach of routine endoscopy. Enteroscopy can now visualize the small intestine, but enteroscopes differ, either visualizing only the upper portion of the jejunum or, in a prolonged procedure, more of the small intestine to the ileum. However, this technique is not widely used.
- Barium studies of the small intestine are difficult to interpret and lack sensitivity.

The development of wireless capsule endoscopy has made the investigation of small-intestinal bleeding easier and more convenient for the patient.

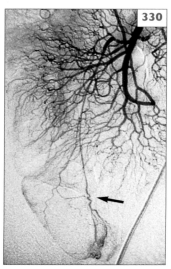

330 Angiogram outlining a Meckel's diverticulum, fed by a long aberrant vessel (arrowed).

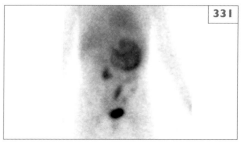

331 Meckel's scan (anterior, 20–25 mins postinjection). There is uptake in the stomach and at the same time by ectopic gastric muosa in the Meckel's diverticulum. (The bladder is also seen due to urinary excretion of the tracer.)

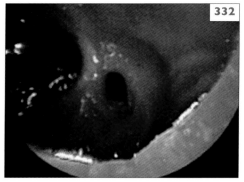

332 Wireless capsule endoscopy showing ulceration on the lip of a Meckel's diverticulum.

Miscellaneous conditions

Constipation may reflect lifestyle or disease

Ascites may reflect hepatic, cardiac, renal, intestinal, or primary peritoneal disease

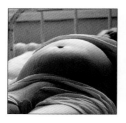
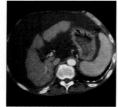
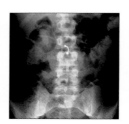
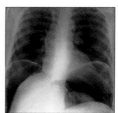

Ascites

Definition

Ascites is defined as the accumulation of fluid in the peritoneal cavity (**333–335**). Such accumulation occurs due to one or more of:

- Local exudation from the peritoneum.
- Hypoproteinaemia.
- High pressure in the portal or systemic venous systems.

Causes

The causes of ascites may reflect local or general problems.

General problems

- Liver failure. This is the commonest cause in clinical practice and is associated with a high mortality within 2 years. Cirrhotic patients in whom ascites develops should be assessed for liver transplantation.
- Cardiac failure/constrictive pericarditis (associated with peripheral oedema and elevated jugular venous pressure).
- Renal failure (associated with marked urinary protein loss).
- Low protein states, e.g. kwashiorkor (protein malnutrition) or PLE.

Local problems

- Peritoneal exudation, e.g. tuberculous peritonitis.
- Peritoneal malignancy: primary – mesothelioma (suspect also asbestos exposure); secondary adenocarcinoma (commonly ovarian, also colon, stomach, or pancreas).

Investigations

- Exclude renal and cardiac causes by examination of jugular venous pressure and urine (consider echocardiogram).
- Exclude gynaecological malignancy (pelvic examination and consider transvaginal ultrasound).
- Examine for stigmata of chronic liver disease.
- Abdominal ultrasound – look for evidence of chronic liver disease (abnormal liver, splenomegaly, abnormal collaterals). Ultrasound is the most sensitive means of detecting small volumes of ascites, as well as pelvic and other malignancy.
- Diagnostic paracentesis – examine for

appearances (blood suggests malignancy, including hepatoma) and protein concentration. The former distinction into transudate (<20 g/l protein) and exudate (>30 g/l) – used to suggest cirrhosis (low protein) or infection (high protein) – has been replaced by consideration of the albumin serum–ascites gradient (*Table 5*). Cytology and culture – a polymorphonuclear leucocyte count

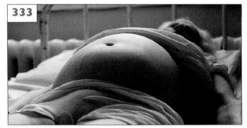

333 Ascites.

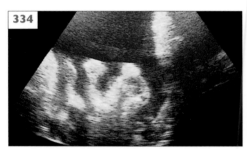

334 Ascites. The ultrasound shows the appearance of loops of bowel floating in echo-free ascitic fluid.

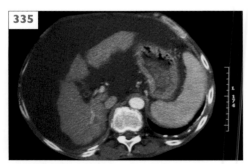

335 Ascites – CT.

exceeding 250×10^6 / l in the ascitic fluid suggests infection (compare peripheral blood counts of polymorphonuclear leucocyte $4,000 - 9,000 \times 10^6$ / l), this is particularly likely to occur when ascites is a complication of hepatic disease. Amylase should be assayed if there is a suspicion of pancreatic ascites.

- CT demonstrates liver outline and liver tumours, alterations in mesentery and peritoneum, and pelvic malignancy (there can be false positives in this area).
- Laparoscopy/peritoneal biopsy.

Management

Reverse precipitating causes if possible. In liver disease (cirrhosis), dietary salt should be restricted. Diuretics should be used judiciously; only 750 ml of ascitic fluid can be reabsorbed spontaneously from the peritoneal cavity, and so a steady weight loss of >0.75 kg/day, in the absence of peripheral oedema, may initiate hypovolaemia. Spironolactone is the first line and can be increased to a dosage of 400 mg/day with a loop diuretic in addition. Hyponatraemia frequently complicates the ascites of chronic liver disease. Diuretics should be used with caution in those with hyponatraemia, and in those with poor renal function.

Large-volume paracentesis (6 l/day) with replacement of albumin (6–8 g/l of ascites), leads to rapid mobilization of ascites in liver disease, and in those refractory to diuretic treatment. TIPSS (see Chapter 9) is an effective treatment for resistant ascites as it reduces portal pressure.

SPONTANEOUS BACTERIAL PERITONITIS

This is a complication of pre-existing ascites, particularly in cirrhotic patients, and is due to the passage of bacteria through the gut wall in the absence of frank perforation. The condition should be considered if a patient with cirrhosis and ascites deteriorates nonspecifically. Patients can be asymptomatic, or present febrile with abdominal pain. Investigation is by paracentesis, and there is an elevated white cell count ($>250 \times 10^6$/l polymorphonuclear leukocytes) in the ascites. Cultures of ascitic fluid in blood culture bottles will frequently identify an organism. Increasing recognition and prompt treatment has reduced the mortality of this condition. Treatment is with broad-spectrum antibiotics; albumin infusion will benefit those with impending hepatorenal failure. Survivors should be considered for liver transplantation and, as recurrent infection is frequent, they should receive prophylactic oral ciprofloxacin or norfloxacin.

TUBERCULOUS PERITONITIS

This condition presents with a doughy abdomen and high-protein ascites (**178**), with lymphocyte predominance. Acid-fast bacilli are often not cultured. Laparoscopy may help in the diagnosis, as can a therapeutic trial of antituberculosis treatment.

Table 5 Causes of ascites – graduated according to whether the gradient of albumin concentration between serum and ascites is high or low

High-gradient ascites Gradient >11 g/l	Low-gradient ascites Gradient <11 g/l
Cirrhosis	Peritoneal carcinomatosis
Alcoholic hepatitis	Tuberculosis peritonitis
Cardiac ascites	Pancreatic ascites
Massive metastases	Biliary ascites
Fulminant hepatic failure	Nephrotic syndrome
Budd–Chiari syndrome	Serositis
Veno-occlusive disease	
Fatty liver	
Myxoedema	

Constipation

Definition

It is essential to find out what the patient means by constipation. Absolute constipation is defined as the failure to pass any stool. If this is associated with pain and distension, then bowel obstruction must be suspected. Otherwise, constipation generally means infrequent passage of stools (normal frequency varies between three times daily to every 3 days). Patients may also use the term to describe the passage of very hard stools, even with normal frequency (**336**). In this case, constipation is usually associated with unproductive efforts to defaecate; a feeling of incomplete evacuation and straining feature in some definitions.

The prevalence of self-reported constipation is very high. In the elderly, severe constipation and straining may be associated with rectal prolapse.

Constipation is a symptom; the causes are broad and encompass lifestyle factors through to major illnesses. Some factors associated with constipation include:

- Inadequate food intake.
- Lack of exercise (profound immobility, e.g. multiple sclerosis, age).
- Lack of roughage (undigested vegetable matter).

Constipation is a feature of a number of colonic and rectal conditions, including cancers, strictures from other causes such as colonic diverticular disease (narrow sigmoid due to muscle hypertrophy), and anal conditions such as fissures.

Various endocrine and metabolic syndromes are also associated with constipation. These include hypercalcaemia, hypokalaemia and hypothyroidism.

Many commonly prescribed drugs, including opiates, anticholinergics, calcium channel blockers, and iron can contribute to constipation.

Special causes

Slow transit constipation

This refers to constipation when slow transit of material from proximal to distal bowel is held to be the key element. Chronic idiopathic slow transit constipation is more frequently diagnosed in women. Colonic transit studies are rarely used in the assessment, although a radiological marker (Shapes test) is occasionally useful.

Pelvic floor disorders

Normal (or only slightly slowed) transit with failure of rectal evacuation occurs in pelvic floor dysfunction. It is suggested by a history of excessive straining to defaecate, and difficulty in evacuating even soft or fluid stools. Sometimes, there is a history of perineal pressure or vaginal digitation to facilitate evacuation. Examination in these instances can reveal perineal descent.

Hirschsprung's disease

This is a congenital disorder, caused by segmental lack of ganglions in the intrinsic neuronal plexuses. The affected segment fails to relax and has no peristalsis, which leads to constipation and proximal colonic dilatation (see Chapter 8).

Treatment

Treatment of constipation is dictated by the underlying cause. Many patients can be adequately managed with minimal investigation and simple measures. This will include advice regarding exercise, increasing fluid, and dietary changes.

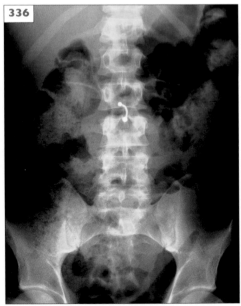

336 Plain abdominal X-ray showing mottled accumulation of faecal matter in ascending colon.

Initially, organic causes should be excluded. Middle-aged or elderly patients presenting with new-onset constipation require some investigation to ensure that they do not have cancer, and have a structurally normal bowel. This could be by barium enema or colonoscopy. This is not always needed, particularly in young patients and patients with a long-standing history of nonprogressive disease.

Use of laxatives

Osmotic laxatives (lactulose, magnesium salts) are preferable to stimulant laxatives (e.g. senna), as prolonged use of stimulant laxatives leads to the destruction of nerve ganglia.

Faecal incontinence

Definition

Faecal incontinence is defined as the involuntary passage of faecal matter, and has a variety of causes. It is a prevalent and distressing symptom among those with diarrhoea, but is frequently unreported by patients. Incontinence occurs only rarely in irritable bowel syndrome or in hormone-mediated diarrhoea. In the elderly, severe constipation can lead to 'overflow incontinence', with the passage of liquid stools forced past obvious hard faeces in the rectum. In this situation, the symptom can be misinterpreted as diarrhoea.

Causes

The causes of incontinence are usually suggested by the history, and include:

- Acute diarrhoeal states, e.g. gastroenteritis.
- Colonic motility abnormalities, e.g. extreme fright.
- Anal sphincter dysfunction. This occurs mainly in elderly patients, but also occasionally in those with severe perianal Crohn's disease, or after injudicious surgery for perianal fistulae.
- Neurological problems – pressure on the spinal cord (this is generally associated with urinary sphincter abnormality).
- Obstetric injury. Sphincter and nerve injury during labour is a common cause of faecal incontinence in women. Frequently there is a history of perineal tear, prolonged labour, or forceps delivery.

Laboratory and special examinations

Many patients can be managed without recourse to specialized investigations.

Anorectal manometry

Pressures in the internal and external sphincters are measured at rest and during squeeze. Rectal sensation and compliance is assessed with incremental inflation of a rectal balloon.

Endoanal ultrasound

The physical integrity of the sphincters can be assessed. This is particularly useful when sphincter trauma is suspected, as muscle defects can be directly visualized.

Management

The management of incontinence is directed to the underlying cause. Symptomatic approaches include:

Stool bulking agents – a solid stool will be better controlled than a liquid stool. Antidiarrhoeal and anticholinergic drugs are helpful.

Surgical repair is appropriate for some patients with discrete sphincter injury.

Acute peritonitis

Definition
This is inflammation of the peritoneum, associated with pain and tenderness when the parietal peritoneum is inflamed. The condition gives local signs, e.g. tenderness over an inflamed appendix. A perforated gut generally leads to generalized peritonitis (classically perforated duodenal ulcer) and causes board-like rigidity of the abdomen. Perforation may, however, be localized (e.g. from colonic diverticula), giving only localized tenderness.

Investigations
Typically, the white cell count will be elevated. A plain radiograph may show free air if the peritonitis was precipitated by perforation (**337**). Serum amylase levels will be markedly increased in acute pancreatitis; when very severe, this can give rise to generalized peritonitis. However, perforation of the upper gastrointestinal tract can moderately elevate serum amylase (loss of amylase-rich fluid from the duodenum into the peritoneum, and hence into the circulation).

Management
Rapid resuscitation is important (marked loss of fluid and protein into the peritoneal cavity will induce hypovolaemia). Generally, urgent surgical intervention is appropriate. Antibiotic therapy should be for wide coverage, including Gram-negative anaerobes.

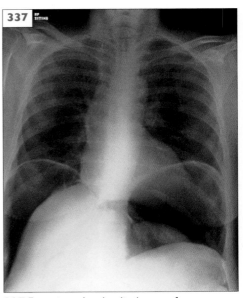

337 Free air under the diaphragm after perforation of the gut.

Appendix

Causes of abdominal pain

Causes of dysphagia

Major gastrointestinal causes of anaemia

Causes of acute gastrointestinal bleeding

Causes of protein-losing enteropathy (PLE)

Causes of abnormal small-intestinal biopsies with villous abnormalities causing malabsorption in adults

Causes of constipation

Screening blood tests for gastrointestinal disease

Causes of diarrhoea and malabsorption

Anatomical investigations and potential value in chronic diarrhoea and malabsorption

Normal ranges, urine (values per 24-hr excretion)

Normal ranges, faeces (values per 24-hr excretion)

Normal ranges, plasma/serum

Gastric function tests – gastric acid secretion (mmol/hr)

Tests for malabsorption

Table 6 Causes of abdominal pain

Gastroduodenal disorders

Nonulcer dyspepsia

Peptic ulcer

Acute gastritis

Tumours

Biliary disorders

Gallstones

Acute cholecystitis

Biliary colic

Hepatic causes

Hepatic congestion (cardiac failure, hepatic venous congestion)

Acute hepatitis

Hepatic tumours

Pancreatic causes

Acute pancreatitis

Chronic pancreatitis

Pancreatic carcinoma

Pseudocysts

Abscesses

Small-intestinal disorders

Motility disorders – irritable bowel

Ischaemic gut

Inflammatory bowel disease

Obstruction

Pseudo-obstruction

Colonic disorders

Motility disorders – irritable bowel, cathartic colon

Diverticulitis

Obstruction

Pericolic abscess

Ischaemic bowel

Miscellaneous

Lead poisoning

Tabes dorsalis

Central

Porphyria

Table 7 Causes of dysphagia

Central

Bulbar palsy

Psedobulbar palsy

Globus hystericus

Local oral

Ulcerative stomatitis

Painful glossitis

Dental problems

Pharyngeal

Muscular weakness/incoordination

Pharyngeal pouch

Extrinsic compression (tumours, lymphadenopathy, etc.)

Oesophageal

Muscular incoordination

    Achalasia

    Spasm

    Systemic sclerosis

    Presby-oesophagus

Webs

Benign strictures

Malignant strictures

Extrinsic compression

Table 8 Major gastrointestinal causes of anaemia

Iron deficiency

Chronic bleeding – NSAIDs treatment, peptic ulcer

Oesophagitis, inflammatory bowel disease, adenomas, carcinomas

Malabsorptive states

Postgastrectomy

Dietary inadequacy

Folate deficiency

Malabsorptive states

Inflammatory bowel disease

Dietary inadequacy

Vitamin B$_{12}$ deficiency

Atrophic gastritis (pernicious anaemia)

Postgastrectomy

Ileal disease and resection

Bacterial overgrowth

Pancreatic disease

Strict vegetarianism

Anaemia of chronic disease

Inflammatory bowel disease

Disseminated malignancy

Acute blood loss

Gastrointestinal bleeding

Table 9 Causes of acute gastrointestinal bleeding

Upper gastrointestinal causes

Common

Gastric and duodenal erosions

Peptic ulcer

Mallory–Weiss tear

Oesophageal varices

Less common

Oesophageal ulcers/oesophagitis

Gastric tumours

Vascular anomalies

Lower gastrointestinal causes

Haemorrhoids

Diverticular bleeding

Inflammatory bowel disease

Adenomas

Carcinomas

Ischaemic colitis

Angiodysplasia

Meckel's diverticulum

Intussusception

Less common (both upper and lower)

Vasculitis

Bleeding disorders

Small-bowel tumours

Small-bowel angiomas

Pseudoxanthoma elasticum

Ehlers–Danlos syndrome

Table 10 Causes of protein-losing enteropathy (PLE)

Primary lymphangiectasia
Secondary lymphangiectasia
Giant rugal hypertrophy of stomach (Ménétrier's)
Zollinger–Ellison syndrome
Inflammatory bowel disease
Carcinomas
Constrictive pericarditis
Whipple's disease
Coeliac disease
Ulcerative ileojejunitis

Table 11 Causes of abnormal small-intestinal biopsies with villous abnormalities causing malabsorption in adults

Coeliac disease
Dermatitis herpetiformis
Ulcerative ileojejunitis
Whipple's disease
Immunodeficiency
Lymphoma
Crohn's disease
Severe radiation enteritis
Graft versus host disease

Table 12 Causes of constipation

Inadequate dietary intake
Inadequate roughage (dietary fibre)
Immobility
Obstructing lesions in bowel
Ileus and pseudo-obstruction
Purgative abuse (cathartic colon)
Pregnancy
Depression
Drugs (opiates, anticholinergics, beta blockers, calcium- and aluminium-containing antacids, etc.)
Paraplegia
Hirschsprung's disease
Metabolic causes (myxoedema, low potassium, hypercalcaemia)

Table 13 Screening blood tests for gastrointestinal disease

Full blood count
Biochemical profile
ESR
CRP
Serum iron and iron-binding capacity
Serum folate and vitamin B_{12}
Suspected malabsorption – add:
   Immunoglobulins
   Endomysial antibody (anti TTG)
Consider HIV testing

Table 14 Causes of diarrhoea and malabsorption

Gastric causes

Postgastrectomy

Gastrinoma – Zollinger–Ellison syndrome

Postvagotomy

Achlorhydria, predisposing to bacterial overgrowth

Gastroenteric fistulae and gastroenterostomy

Pancreatic causes

Chronic pancreatitis

Pancreatic resection

Carcinoma

Cystic fibrosis

Schwachman's syndrome

Congenital enzyme deficiency

Hepatobiliary causes

Cholestasis

Bile-salt therapy

Small-intestinal causes

Short gut syndrome

Ileal resection

Lactase deficiency

Coeliac disease

Dermatitis herpetiformis

Ulcerative ileojejunitis

Tropical sprue

Postinfectious malabsorption

Whipple's disease

Lymphangiectasia

Lymphoma

Bacterial overgrowth

Infections – viral, bacterial, protozoal

Immunodeficiency, including AIDS

Radiation enteritis

Food allergies

Eosinophilic enteritis

Mesenteric ischaemia

Vasculitis

Abetalipoproteinaemia

Amyloidosis

Autonomic neuropathy

Visceral myopathy

Graft versus host disease

Systemic sclerosis

Enterocolic fistula

Colonic causes

Colonic resection

Infections

Ulcerative colitis

Crohn's disease

Irritable bowel

Diverticular disease

Pseudomembranous colitis

Constipation with overflow

Microscopic colitis

Collagenous colitis

Radiation colitis

Purgative abuse (cathartic colon)

Villous adenoma

Carcinoma

Graft versus host disease

Endocrine causes

Diabetes

Carcinoid syndrome

VIPoma

Thyrotoxicosis

Addison's disease

Zollinger–Ellison syndrome

Medullary carcinoma of thyroid

Drugs

Very many – magnesium-containing antacids, antibiotics, purgatives, cytotoxics, etc.

Sorbitol as artificial sweetener

Table 15 Anatomical investigations and potential value in chronic diarrhoea and malabsorption

Endoscopic duodenal/jejunal biopsy

Coeliac disease
Tropical sprue
Lymphoma
Whipple's disease
Alpha-chain disease
Giardiasis
HIV enteropathy
Mycobacterium avium intracellulare
Lymphangiectasia
Kaposi's sarcoma

Small-intestinal radiology

Malabsorptive pattern
Crohn's disease
Jejunal diverticulosis
Lymphangiectasia
Lymphoma
Blind loops
Resection
Enteroenteric connections
Pseudo-obstruction
Strictures
Tuberculosis
Whipple's disease
Nodular lymphoid hyperplasia

Sigmoidoscopy, colonoscopy, and biopsy

Ulcerative colitis
Crohn's disease
Diverticulitis
Minimal change and collagenous colitis
Melanosis coli
Amoebiasis
Amyloidosis
Lymphoma
Carcinoma

Barium enema

Carcinoma
Ulcerative colitis
Crohn's disease
Diverticular disease
Ischaemic colitis
Cathartic colon
Fistula
Tuberculosis

ERCP

Chronic pancreatitis
Cancer of pancreas
Cholestatic liver disease

NORMAL RANGES

Note: All normal ranges should be checked against local laboratory reference ranges. This applies to all tests, but is particularly important for dynamic tests (e.g. acid secretion) and immunoassays.

Table 16 Normal ranges, urine (values per 24-hr excretion)

Constituent	SI or other International units	Traditional units
Amino acid nitrogen-free	4–20 mmol	50–300 mg
Amylase	200–1,500 U	10–7,000 Henry–Chiamori units
Calcium	2.5–7.5 mmol	100–300 mg
Copper	0.2–1.5 μmol	10–100 μg
Creatinine	9–18 mmol	1.0–2.0 g
Glucose	0.1–1.0 mmol	20–200 mg
5-Hydroxyindoleacetic acid	10–45 μmol	2–8 mg
Indicans	0.1–0.4 mmol	20–80 mg
Lead	0–0.3 μmol	0–60 μg
Nitrogen – total	0.7–1.5 mol	10–20 g
Osmolality	700–1,500 mmol	700–1,500 mosmol
Phosphate	15–50 mmol	0.5–1.5 g
Porphyrins		
δ-Aminolaevulinic acid	1–40 μmol	0.1–5.0 mg
Porphobilinogen	1–12 μmol	0.2–2.0 mg
Coproporphyrin	0.15–0.3 μmol	100–200 μg
Uroporphyrin	6–40 nmol	5–30 μg
Potassium	40–120 mmol	40–120 mEq
Protein – total	40–120 mg	40–120 mg
Sodium	100–250 mmol	100–250 mEq

Table 17 Normal ranges, faeces (values per 24-hr excretion)

Constituent	SI or other International units	Traditional units
Total wet weight	60–250 g	60–250 g
Total dry weight	20–60 g	20–60 g
Fat – total	10–18 mmol	3–5 g
Nitrogen – total	70–110 mmol	1–1.5 g

Table 18 Normal ranges, plasma/serum

Constituent	SI or other international units	Traditional units
Amino acid nitrogen	2.5–4.0 mmol/l	3.5–5.5 mg/100 ml
Ammonia (whole blood)	12–60 µmol/l	20–100 µg/100 ml
Amylase	70–300 U/l	40–160 Somogyi units/100 ml
Anion gap	6–16 mmol/l	6–16 mEq/l
Bicarbonate	24–30 mmol/l	24–30 mEq/l
Bilirubin		
Total	5.0–17 µmol/l	0.3–1.0 mg/100 ml
Conjugated	<3.0 µmol/l	<0.2 mg/100 ml
Caeruloplasmin	0.3–0.6 g/l	30–60 mg/100 ml
Calcium	2.1–2.6 mmol/l	8.5–10.5 mg/l00 ml
Carbon dioxide (whole blood)	4.5–6.0 kPa	35–46 mmHg
Carbonic acid	1.1–1.4 mmol/l	1.1–1.4 mEq/l
Carotenoids	1.0–5.5 µmol/l	50–300 µg/100 ml
Chloride	95–105 mmol/l	95–105 mEq/l
Cholesterol – total	4.0–6.5 mmol/l	160–260 mg/100 ml
Copper	13–24 µmol/l	80–150 µg/100 ml
Cortisol	200–700 nmol/l	8–35 µg/100 ml
Creatine kinase	3–150 U/l	3–150 IU/l
Creatinine	60–120 µmol/l	0.7–1.4 mg/100 ml
Fatty acids – free	0.3–0.6 mmol/l	0.3–0.6 mEq/l
Ferritin	15–250 µg/l	1.5–25 µg/100 ml
Folate	5.0–20 µg/l	5.0–20 ng/ml
Gastrin	5–50 pmol/l	10–100 pg/ml
Glucose (whole blood)		
Venous	3.0–5.0 mmol/l	55–90 mg/100 ml
Capillary	3.2–5.2 mmol/l	60–95 mg/100 ml
γ-Glutamyltransferase	5–45 U/l	5–45 IU/l
Haptoglobins	5–30 µmol/l	30–180 mg/100 ml
Iron	11–34 µmol/l	60–190 µg/100 ml
Iron-binding capacity – total	45–75 µmol/l	250–400 µg/100 ml
Ketones	0.06–0.2 mmol/l	0.06–0.2 mEq/l
Lactate	0.75–2.0 mmol/l	0.75–2.0 mEq/l
Lead (whole blood)	0.5–1.7 µmol/l	10–35 µg/100 ml

Table 19 Normal ranges, plasma/serum (contd)

Lipase	18–280 U/l	0–1.5 Cherry–Crandall units
Lipids – total fasting	4.5–10 g/l	450–1000 mg/100 ml
Magnesium	0.7–1.0 mmol/l	1.8–2.4 mg/100 ml
5'-Nucleotidase	2–15 U/l	2–15 IU/l
Osmolality	275–295 mmol/kg	275–295 mosmol/kg
Oxygen (whole blood)	11–15 kPa	85–105 mmHg
pH	7.36–7.42	7.36–7.42
Phosphatases		
Total acid	0.5–5.5 U/l	0.3–3.0 KAu/100 ml
'Prostatic' acid	0–1 U/l	0–0.5 KAu/100 ml
Total alkaline	20–95 U/l	3–13 KAu/100 ml
Phosphate – inorganic	0.8–1.4 mmol/l	2.5–4.5 mg/100 ml
Phospholipids	1.8–3.0 mmol/l	150–250 mg/100 ml
Potassium	3.5–5.0 mmol/l	3.5–5.0 mEq/l
Protein		
Total	60–80 g/l	6.0–8.0 g/100 ml
Albumin	35–50 g/l	3.5–5.0 g/100 ml
Globulin – total	18–32 g/l	1.8–3.2 g/100 ml
γ-Globulin – total	7–15 g/l	0.7–1.5 g 100 ml
IgA	1.0–4.0 g/l	100–400 mg/100 ml
IgG	8.0–16.0 g/l	800–1600 mg/100 ml
IgM	0.5–2.5 g/l	50–250 mg/100 ml
Fibrinogen	2–4 g/l	0.2–0.4 g/100 ml
Sodium	135–145 mmol/l	135–145 mEq/l
Transaminases		
Alanine	5–25 U/l	5–25 IU/l
Aspartate	5–35 U/l	5–35 IU/l
Transferrin	1.2–2.0 g/l	120–200 mg/100 ml
Triglyceride	0.3–1.8 mmol/l	25–150 mg/100 ml
Trypsin	140–400 µg/l	140–400 ng/ml
Urea	3.0–6.5 mmol/l	18–40 mg/100 ml
Urate	0.1–0.4 mmol/l	1.5–7.0 mg/100 ml
VIP	<5 pmol/l	
Vitamin A	1.0–3.0 µmol/l	30–90 µg/100 ml
Vitamin B$_{12}$	160–900 ng/l	160–900 pg/ml
Vitamin D	8–60 nmol/l	3–4 ng/ml
Zinc	12–17 µmol/l	80–110 µg/100 ml

DYNAMIC TESTS

Table 20 Gastric function tests – gastric acid secretion (mmol/hr)

Ulcer	Normal Basal	Peak	Duodenal Basal	Peak
Men	1 (0–5)	22 (1–45)	4 (0–15)	42 (15–100)
Women	1 (0–5)	12 (1–30)	2 (0–5)	32 (15–100)

	Zollinger–Ellison syndrome Basal	Peak
Typical	15–30	60–120

Note: The significant difference noted in Zollinger–Ellison syndrome is high basal, as well as high peak, gastric acid output. Zollinger–Ellison syndrome also has high fasting gastrin (>60 pg/ml) – this should be tested when patients have been off acid-suppressant drugs for adequate time (days to weeks), as achlorhydria also gives high gastrin levels.

Table 21 Tests for malabsorption

Fat

3-day faecal fat >18 mmol or 6 g fat per day when on 70 g fat intake

Carbohydrate – xylose tolerance test

Typically 25 g oral xylose

>25% ingested dose after 6 hr in urine (note: this requires normal renal function)

1- or 2-hr blood estimations may be performed

Lactose tolerance test

This tests for disaccharidase deficiency and should normally show a rise in blood glucose of 20 mg/dl after 50 g lactose

Clinically, whether this provokes symptoms of diarrhoea and flatulence is also helpful

Pancreatic function testing

1. PABA test: >50% ingested PABA (500–1.5 g orally) in urine over 6 hr (note: this requires normal renal function)
2. Pancreolauryl secretion: >30% ingested dose in urine over 6 hr

Index